Optimizing Emergency Department Throughput

Operations Management Solutions
for Health Care Decision Makers

"Much as a surgeon uses a scapel, retractor and other tools, to operate on a patient, Shiver (or Optimizing ED Throughput) gives the healthcare manager the tools they need to enhance the function of the Emergency Department, the "front door" of every community's health care system. The text is clear, concise and understandable to those lacking a technical background but who still want to apply fairly sophisticated techniques to improving the patient experience and the productivity of ED staff."

J. Knox Singleton
President and CEO
Inova Health System

"Optimizing Emergency Department Throughput is a breakthrough in creating a framework for ED transformation. It uses state-of-the-art improvement techniques to solve problems bedeviling America: crowding and delays in critical treatment. Shiver and Eitel offer clear, practical approaches that leaders can use to get results."

Bruce Siegel MD MPH
Director
Center for Health Care Quality
Department of Health Policy

"For those physician leaders and hospital administrators who wonder if there are solutions out there for their frustrating overcrowding and flow issues, this book provides a needed introduction to the science of reengineering your health care delivery system. The authors build on decades of experience together with proven models from the literature that will help you move your organization forward, while improving patient and staff satisfaction."

Christopher MB Fernandes,
Professor of Emergency Medicine,
University of Western Ontario/Chair, Medical Advisory Committee,
London Health Sciences Centre, London, Ontario.

"This is a very practical, idea filled book that should be read by any healthcare professional supervising, dependent upon, working in or "sinking" in one of America's besieged emergency departments. I found myself repeatedly circling, underlining, and writing in the margins throughout the book. In the introduction, Shiver reports that ED's "are not at a tripping point; they are at a breaking point". The "tools" presented in this book can prevent or at least delay your tumble into that seemingly inevitable abyss."

Robert J. Cates MS, MD
Chairman of Emergency Medicine
Inova Fairfax Hospital

"Because the ED is a major gateway to all hospital services, a public health asset, and an economic driver or millstone, *Optimizing Emergency Department Throughput* is an essential read for all CNEs, COOs and CEOs."

Lawrence L. White, Jr. MHA, FACHE
Research Assistant Professor
School of Public and Community Health Sciences
The University of Montana

"Shiver and Eitel have provided a valuable primer for all who recognize the ED as the front door to the hospital and who want to assure an efficient and effective journey beyond that door."

Mark Parrington, FACHE
Vice President, Strategic Transactions
Catholic Health Initiatives

Optimizing Emergency Department Throughput

Operations Management Solutions for Health Care Decision Makers

John M. Shiver, MHA, LFACHE, FAAMA

David Eitel, MD, MBA

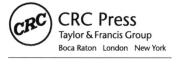

CRC Press
Taylor & Francis Group
Boca Raton   London   New York

CRC Press is an imprint of the
Taylor & Francis Group, an **informa** business

A PRODUCTIVITY PRESS BOOK

Productivity Press
Taylor & Francis Group
270 Madison Avenue
New York, NY 10016

© 2010 by Taylor and Francis Group, LLC
Productivity Press is an imprint of Taylor & Francis Group, an Informa business

International Standard Book Number: 978-1-4200-8377-4 (Paperback)

Library of Congress Cataloging-in-Publication Data

Optimizing emergency department throughput : Operations Management Solutions for Health Care Decision Makers / editors, John M. Shiver and David Eitel.
    p. ; cm.
   Includes bibliographical references and index.
   ISBN 978-1-4200-8377-4 (papercover : alk. paper)
    1. Hospitals--Emergency services--Management. I. Shiver, John M. II. Eitel, David. III. Title.
   [DNLM: 1. Emergency Service, Hospital--organization & administration. 2. Efficiency, Organizational. 3. Models, Organizational.
 4. Quality Assurance, Health Care. W X 215 O615 2010]

RA975.5.E5O677 2010
362.11068--dc22
                                                                                            2009026910

Visit the Taylor & Francis Web site at
http://www.taylorandfrancis.com

and the Productivity Press Web site at
http://www.productivitypress.com

Contents

Introduction: Description of Current Status of Emergency Departments and Hospitals

According to a June 2006 report issued by the Institute of Medicine of the Academy of Science, the emergency medical system in America is in critical condition. Across the country ambulances are turned away from emergency departments (EDs) and patients are waiting hours and sometimes days to be admitted to a hospital room. Hospitals are finding it hard to get specialist physicians to come to treat emergency patients.[1] Our emergency medical system is at a stage where it cannot support the public's demand for care.

In the decade leading up to 2006 the country saw the annual number of visits to EDs rise by 32% to 119.2 million visits. This equates to an annual increase of 3.2%.[2] Like economic inflation, society's need for medical attention is eating into our medical wealth at a rate that cannot be sustained. Making the situation worse in the same period that utilization was increasing markedly, the number of EDs available to meet this growing need fell from 4,019 to 3,833. Adding to the stress, the number of visits per person increased by 18% from 34.2/100 people to 40.5/100. So, not only is the absolute number of visits rising and places to treat this growing demand falling, but society is using the service more frequently. We are more dependent upon this resource as a society than ever before and the pressure is growing.

A common discussion among ED professionals is the perception that many patients are not really emergency patients and could be treated in another setting at another time. A National Center for Health Statistics report supports this in that only 10.8% of visits are truly emergent (needing to be seen within 1 to 14 minutes).[2] However, another 36.6% are urgent (needing to be seen within 15 minutes to an hour). Semi-urgent patients (needing to be seen within 1 to 2 hours) represent 22% of all patients seen in EDs nationally. Nonurgent and unclassified represent the remainder, about 30% of visits. In other words, over half of all patients presenting for care in EDs could indeed be treated in alternative settings and arguably for less cost and in shorter time. Over the years these numbers

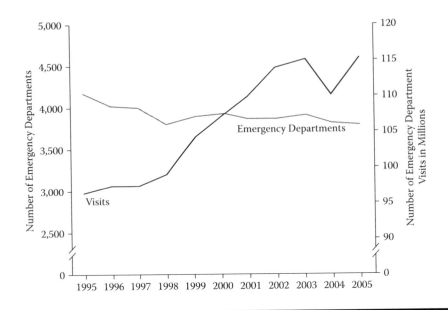

Figure 0.1   National Hospital Ambulatory Medical Survey, American Hospital Association. Sources: CDC/NCHS.

have generated an ongoing discussion of how to redirect patients. This topic is discussed later in the book.

Although the majority of patients waited less than an hour to see a physician (61.8%), the median patient care time was 2.6 hours. Between 1997 and 2004, the median wait time for heart attack patients increased 150 percent from 8 minutes to 20 minutes.[3] We all have examples among family and friends that fall well outside these averages. Again, that is only the average.

The time of arrival in EDs is a much studied and discussed issue. Nationally, the lowest patient volume is seen in the early morning (5 a.m. to 6 a.m.), while the highest volumes are seen in the early evening between 6 p.m. and 9 p.m. The difference between these times is about a multiple of 3. This is probably no surprise to anyone involved in the business, as it seems to correlate closely with our lifestyles. People are occupied with school and work during the day and may seek care at more convenient times. It also correlates closely with the availability of traditional physician office hours. In fact, EDs provide about 11% of all ambulatory care in the country, which is interesting given that emergency physicians represent only 3.3% of all active physicians.

Nationwide, EDs are under growing pressure to treat more patients in fewer facilities resulting in overcrowding, patients waiting to be seen, patients lying on gurneys for hours waiting for discharge, and patients boarding in hallways awaiting inpatient beds. While these patients are being subjected to long waits, hospitals are consuming very expensive resources in an inefficient manner. Not to make too fine a point of it, we have all read the horror stories of patients dying awaiting care.

The financial condition of hospital EDs is a hot topic among managers in many hospitals. The uninsured represent 17.3% of all patients treated in EDs nationally but this varies greatly by individual facilities. The largest percentage of patients, at 39.7%, have private insurance, while Medicaid and State Children's Health Insurance Program (SCHIP) covers 25.5% and Medicare covers 17.3%.

Going forward there does not appear to be a quick solution. And it may get much worse before it gets better. We are facing a massive increase in the number of people who will be classified as elderly. The baby boomer population will be entering the market as elderly beginning in 2011. Already the percentage of people being seen in EDs and classified as immediate or urgent is at 24.6%. This can only be expected to increase the stress on EDs as more acute patients enter the system.

All of this said, a 2003 report authored by Paul Breslin, of Noblis, noted that EDs accounted for the greatest percentage of hospital admissions.[4] EDs also were the largest source of inpatient lab tests (67%) and radiology exams (75%). In the 2006 National Center for Health Statistics report, the percent of admissions was 50.2% nationally.[2] This would indicate that most hospitals are almost totally dependent upon their EDs for their economic survival, regardless of payer mix. Hospitals may wish, from an economic perspective, that the ED would go away, but as a practical matter, it is their lifeline.

In summary, our country's EDs are stressed to the breaking point. Originally, EDs were established to care for the true emergency in an era when health care was much less sophisticated and our society less demanding. As now structured and organized, our EDs today can no longer handle the demands being placed upon them. Our society is demanding care, quality, and service. The health care industry would be naive to believe that there will be help coming from outside to resolve this problem. We can be sure that the external pressures will continue to increase until the pain is so great that we make the changes ourselves or face the consequences.

Focusing on ambulatory care, particularly the ED, is a relatively new phenomenon and requires a paradigm shift in thinking. The specialty of emergency medicine has only been around since the mid-1970s. EDs, as we now know them, are generally less than 40 years old in many communities. Up until now many hospitals considered the ED a necessary community service offered only grudgingly. It is now being recognized as a core service, but one that is structurally flawed having been designed for a different time and market.

Our EDs demand a new way of thinking. They are not at a tipping point; they are at a breaking point. Under current loads and trends they are going to begin to break and these breakdowns will be painful and ultimately dangerous to society.

It is not enough to simply restructure our existing system; we will need to consider a wholesale restructuring of the way ambulatory care is provided with new delivery models and greater use of technological solutions. We must make our existing system more effective. Business as usual will not suffice. Hospitals must make the system function better. This will require the utilization of more scientific methodologies to manage the system and improve efficiencies. It will require a new way of thinking.

Improving efficacy requires change, and change is not a comfortable exercise for either the individual or the organization. Creating an organizational culture that can accept and embrace change is the role of leadership. Leaders must begin the process of creating a culture accepting of change and focused on productivity.

Layered on top of all of this is the fact that EDs are the foci for health care services in the event of a disaster. The terrorist attacks of September 11, 2001, made this entirely too clear. Communities across the country look toward hospitals and their EDs for critical health care services in the event of a pandemic, natural disaster, or terrorist attack. The fragility and lack of capacity are not up to the demands of anything out of the ordinary. The ordinary is breaking them already. Health care leaders must step up to the leadership role and begin addressing how community hospitals will provide critical infrastructure services in the event of an untoward occurrence.

The purpose of this book is to provide health care leaders tools they can utilize to optimize the performance of EDs and thereby improve service to patients, employees, and communities. The techniques described herein can be utilized to quantify improvements, enhance predictability of workflow, and improve staff scheduling. The data derived using these techniques can serve as powerful evidence in support of making change.

—John M. (Jay) Shiver, MHA, LFACHE, FAAMA

References

1. Future of Emergency Care, Institute of Medicine, June 14, 2006, Washington, DC.
2. Pitts, Stephen R., Richard W. Niska, Jianmin Xu, and Catharine W. Burt. August 6, 2008. National Hospital Ambulatory Medical Care Survey: 2006 Emergency Department Summary. National Health Statistics Report, no. 7. Hyattsville, MD: National Center for Health Statistics.
3. Andrew Wilber et al., *Health Affairs*, 2, January 15, 2008.
4. Paul Breslin, *The British Review*, October 2003.

Acknowledgments

I wish to thank my colleagues in the former section of Health Services Design in the Emergency Department at the York Hospital—Dean Johnson, Tom Falvo, Lance Grove, Michael Kleinman, Sueanne McKniff, and David Vega—for their insights and innovations.

—David Eitel

I wish to thank my wife, Debbie, for her support all these years. I would also like to acknowledge the valuable contribution of my mentor, J. Robert MacNaughton, who taught me critical thinking skills.

—John M. Shiver

Chapter 1

Fixing the Front End:
Why Would an Emergency Department Medical Director or Nursing Supervisor Wish to Install Emergency Severity Index (ESI) Triage?

David Eitel and Tom Falvo

Until Emergency Severity Index (ESI) triage became available in the Unites States, emergency department (ED) triage was most commonly performed by ED nurses using a poorly designed, nonstandardized, three-level triage method. Most often the three-level method classified incoming patients as emergent, urgent, or non-urgent; or as a level 1, 2 or 3 patient. These three-level methods hinged greatly on an assessment by the triage nurse of "How long do you think this patient can *wait*?" The reliability of the triage assignments produced by these three-level methods, asking this type of question, was very poor. That is, the inter-rater (between triage nurses) and test–retest (same nurse doing triage again) assignments that these three-level methods produced were very inconsistent. In contradistinction, the definitions used to differentiate patients with ESI five-level triage are explicit and are easily understood—by clinicians and nonclinicians (such as hospital administrators) alike. In ESI triage the ED triage nurse asks two questions: Who should be seen first (levels 1 and 2)? and What do you think the patient will need in terms of resources (where resources are specified) to reach an ED disposition (levels 5, 4, and 3)? The ESI Triage Research Team believes that a principal goal of ED triage should be to determine who should be seen first. But a second major goal of ED triage should be not to just "sort" but to "stream." This second goal of ED triage is about getting the right patient to the right resources in the right place and at the right time. ESI triage is fundamentally rooted in an industrial engineering way of thinking. ESI triage is about *quick sort and stream*; indeed, it is often called the "Quick Sort" step in an emergency department flow mapping or simulation modeling exercise.

So, why would an emergency department medical director or nursing supervisor wish to install ESI triage in his/her ED?

Real-Time Management of Emergency Department (ED) Flow: Streaming and Not Just Sorting

In the hands of trained and experienced ED nursing staff, ESI triage produces a reliable and reproducible classification of incoming patients into one of five actionable categories. The 1s and 2s go into your critical care area. The various types of 3s, like 3-geriatric, can go into areas you have readied for that purpose. The predicted lower resource intensity patients (the level 4s and 5s) could be directed to an alternative treatment area within your department. Using ESI triage offers you an opportunity for the parallel processing of patients and a method of safely unloading your main ED. ESI triage is a tool for distribution, not just sorting, of workloads.

Communicating ED Workload to Others

The definitions used to differentiate patients within the ESI triage algorithm (tool) are explicit, reproducible, and easily understood. The definitions for each ESI triage level can be readily communicated to anyone, including nonclinical hospital administrators.

Example: You are on your way to a meeting where you will be discussing ED staffing needs with your administration, and the very negative effects "overcrowding" is having on patient safety and staff retention. Last evening you had six level 2 patients that had to remain in your waiting room for a total of 6 hours. (The definition of an ESI level 2 patient is: "A high risk situation; the patient is acutely confused/lethargic/disoriented, or in severe pain or distress." Basically, an ESI level 2 assignment means "take right back.") This was of great concern to your competent and motivated staff last night, all of whom felt terrible that they could not provide better patient care. Staff members are contemplating leaving the ED.

Using the common language of the ESI, you and the CEO can have a more meaningful discussion of last evening's ED staffing and related patient care issues.

ESI Case Mix Data and Predictive Management

Example: You have had ESI triage installed for a few months and have therefore been able to collect the following data by ESI triage level:

Triage Level	Case Mix (% Total)	Admit Rate	ED Length of Stay (Hours)
Level 1	125 (2%)	73%	2.4
Level 2	1,756 (22%)	54%	4.0
Level 3	3,173 (39%)	24%	3.4
Level 4	2,197 (27%)	2%	2.0
Level 5	812 (10%)	.003%	1.4
Total	8,063		

What can you determine from this kind of operational data? How might you and the senior hospital managers be able to use this kind of information?

First, because the ED nursing staff are well trained (with regular refresher classes) and follow the ESI algorithm while doing "quick sort" triage, you are confident that the information is reliable.

This data tells you just over half of all of your level 2 patients are being admitted to the hospital. By counting the number of level 2 patients in your ED at any given time, you and the hospital managers can get a good sense of the patient service load that will soon be arriving in inpatient units upstairs. You do not yet know for certain whether a particular patient will be admitted, but by looking at the ESIs of a group of patients you can make a fairly accurate estimate of how many are likely to require an inpatient bed. Further, by tracking the admission destinations of all level 2 patients who arrive at your hospital over a period of time, you could develop destination distribution data that allows you and the hospital management team to proactively prepare for the anticipated service load upstairs, as well as other "downstream demand" as additional laboratory and imaging services are ordered.

Forecasting Demand Combined with "Capacity to Serve" Planning

From your patient registration system you have been able to obtain the time at which every patient arrived in your ED this past year. Your database now includes the rate of incoming broken down by the hour of the day and day of the week for a 12-month period. You can compare the usual service loads on a

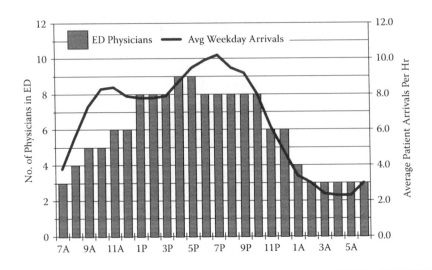

Figure 1.1 York Hospital emergency department physician staffing versus average arrivals on a typical weekday.

typical weekday versus a typical weekend day. This pattern of incoming arrival data looks like the jagged line in Figure 1.1 and Figure 1.2 when graphed.

The pattern of incoming (demand/service load) for all comers is, to your amazement, surprisingly repeatable. In general, most weekday days look like Figure 1.1 and most weekend days look (and feel) like Figure 1.2. It turns out that your ED's service loads by day of week and times of day are actually, contrary to popular belief, very predictable. Sundays begin a lot busier and stay busier. Sundays look like Sundays, and Wednesdays look like Wednesdays. Knowing

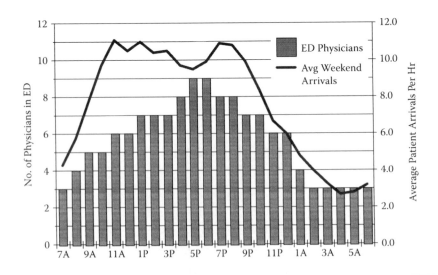

Figure 1.2 York Hospital emergency department physician staffing versus average arrivals on a typical weekend.

this, you can now adjust your staffing accordingly and avoid the safety issues and long waits that are burning out your staff and leading to patient complaints.

However, since you are an operationally insightful medical director with ESI triage installed, you discover that additional data is available. You now have a few months worth of ESI *case mix data*. You can determine the rate of incoming patients by ESI triage level (level 1s, 2s, 3s, etc.) by the hour of the day and day of week. Therefore you can plot out the rate of incoming each hour of the day by ESI level. You, as a sophisticated medical director, can now further fine-tune both your department's staffing pattern and the skills mix that is needed to accommodate level 1 and level 2 traumas and level 3 geriatric nursing home patients. You will be able to do a much better job of *rostering* (scheduling the number and skill levels of your ED staff) according to the hour of the day and day of the week. You have always felt that doing staffing calculations using linear thinking (the math of total volumes and averages) was not cutting it. Now, with ESI case mix data plotted over time, you can use nonlinear thinking to help you out as an ED service unit manager.

Now that you have used ESI triage data to determine your ED's true daily service load, it is time to apply something called statistical forecasting.

Statistical Forecasting

Once ESI triage has been up and running and you have collected ESI case mix data for an extended period of time, you can add statistical forecasting to your management toolset. That means you can use ESI time series case mix data with statistical forecasting methods and forecasting software to predict the ED workloads that would be expected under different scenarios. You will consider building this into a new approach to annual ED forecasting and then budgeting.

Emergency Department Workflow Analysis Including Lean and Six Sigma Improvement Methods

This isn't cost reduction, its process change.

—Lou Giuliani, CEO of ITT

Most major industries now use workflow analysis methods (including Lean and Six Sigma) as tools to help them improve service performance. Workflow analysis begins with "activity sequencing," also known as flow mapping or flowcharting.

Workflow diagramming for the emergency department involves, as you might expect, creating a comprehensive visual display of every step (every activity) patients might experience while navigating their way through the department from the time they first enter until they leave. (This exercise could be done for any service unit in the hospital.)

Once the initial mapping has been completed, it is very important to have the workflow diagram reviewed by and discussed with your frontline staff. This ensures that the diagrams reflect what actually happens to a patient in your department. Your corrected flowchart should now reflect the true as-is state of your operations. It is surprising how much you will learn from this fairly simple but powerful exercise.

Once the true as-is state of your ED has been captured on a flowchart, operational data can be added to make the workflow diagram more useful. Because patients are not all the same, this is where having ESI case mix data allows medical directors to create more accurate and meaningful workflow diagrams.

Documenting the types and numbers of resources and the amount of staff time that is consumed at each step, as well as understanding the probability patterns at each of the decision points in the flow map, significantly increases the flow chart's utility as a collaborative, predictive modeling, and management tool. It allows you to analyze the ED's business processes and determine where in the overall workflow time and money are being expended without adding value to the patient's experience, the definition of waste. This type of analysis is often referred to as "static" or "conceptual" modeling.

Having completed these steps you are now ready to consider adding two business improvement methods to your ED management toolkit: Lean and Six Sigma. A detailed discussion of Lean and Six Sigma methodologies is beyond the scope of this chapter, but each uses a proscriptive approach and a specific set of techniques to improve system performance.

Briefly, Lean (often called process excellence) is a business improvement method that improves the efficiency of work processes, to a large extent through simplification. Removing waste (unnecessary steps, redundancy, excessive paperwork, long waiting times, etc.) frees up resources that can be applied to more useful (value added) work.

The major analysis tool of Lean is something called time value stream mapping, a visual assessment tool that follows easily on the heels of the ED workflow diagramming (conceptual modeling) approach mentioned earlier.

Just so you can say you have heard it once, the five steps of Lean are:

1. Define your customers (clients, patient types) and what they really want.
2. Understand, in detail, the processes you use to deliver care.
3. Streamline the flow of patients through the system.
4. Shift from push to pull.
5. Maintain the gains, monitor progress, and continue to reduce waste.

Lean methodology has been used quite successfully in manufacturing, particularly by the automotive industry. There is now a growing interest in applying these techniques to service industries such as health care. Because service delivery differs in many ways from "making widgets," it is necessary to adapt the Lean methods traditionally used in manufacturing to make them more service oriented.

The tools of Lean thinking are extremely simple to learn and apply. Process excellence (in contrast to Six Sigma) does not require significant quantitative reasoning, mathematical, or statistical skills. It can be taught and understood at a high school educational level. Change management becomes the real issue.

Six Sigma often builds upon the initial work of process excellence with a highly proscriptive approach that applies additional quantitative reasoning to the initial analysis. It requires a higher level of mathematical and statistical skills to implement, and is more capital intensive than the Lean business improvement method. Adopting the Six Sigma approach therefore requires the organization to institute a comprehensive training program and develop experienced facilitators (known as Green and Black Belts) to help out with what are major improvement projects.

Again briefly, and just so you have also heard this at least once, Six Sigma uses the DMAIIC approach:

1. Define
2. Measure
3. Analyze
4. Improve
5. Implement
6. Control

ESI Service Mix Data and Lean-Six Sigma: All Patients Are Not the Same

The Lean and Six Sigma business improvement methods require decision makers to make the leap from their current management style to a process and then systems way of thinking and managing. Both methods emphasize the importance of incorporating accurate operational data and the input of frontline workers into decision making. Both use multidisciplinary teams and project management methods. Either methodology offers a consistent approach for leadership to apply, working closely with its frontline staff, to develop fiscal strategy or initiate systematic business improvement and orderly change.

Because both of these methodologies are strongly data based and ESI triage supplies reliable presenting case mix data about your ED, installing ESI triage allows Lean or Six Sigma to be much more robustly implemented within an ED. In general, health care organizations should have their processes "Leaned" before attempting Six Sigma. Because Lean is not as capital intensive (just the opposite), it is often the ideal choice for a health care organization that is just beginning the journey toward process excellence.

We often compare the adoption of Lean and Six Sigma process excellence methods to emergency physicians incorporating RSI (rapid sequence induction) and intubation into their clinical practices. In contrast to the early years of our specialty when establishing an airway in the ED was often a matter of luck, we are now trained in a proscriptive approach to airway control that includes a specific set of tools and drugs, which are used in a particular order, with flexibility to accommodate variation as problems arise. After training, application, and practice, it is now expected that we will achieve our objective: getting the tube in the right orifice, reliably, quickly, and safely—usually on the first attempt even in the face of great clinical complexity. This is an example of process excellence successfully applied in clinical practice. Perhaps it is time to apply similar methods and determination to the management of ED business practices.

The Institute for Health Improvement (www.ihi.org) recently announced a call to action titled "Going Lean in Health Care." The American Society for Quality (www.asq.org) has also begun a major initiative to introduce quality management methods and Lean Six Sigma training to a new target audience of health care leaders. Even the Healthcare Financial Management Association (www.hfma.org) now includes Lean Six Sigma programs in its seminars. By the time this book is published these terms will most likely be familiar to ED medical directors everywhere. If you have not yet discussed Lean or Six Sigma with your hospital's administrative team, you soon will.

Dynamic Modeling: Simulation Modeling

Finally, with ESI triage installed and reliable ESI case mix data available, a medical director has the opportunity to model his or her ED using a powerful decision support tool called process simulation. Process simulation is used when variation, interdependency, and complexity need to be understood and quantified. Understanding these three important characteristics of any service operation will help you to become a more effective director. Following are some examples to explain variation, interdependency, and complexity.

Variation

If driving to work takes, on average, 15 minutes, we will usually (95 percent of the time) arrive within some time range, let's say between 12 and 18 minutes. It is unusual to arrive exactly 15 minutes after we leave the house. It is also unlikely to take us 2 hours. Much of the variation in each day's drive is (or could be) predicted in advance, if we simply tracked the time data for departure and arrival.

If it is possible to do that in regular life, then why can you not predict variations in the times that the nursing staff and technicians complete different patient care activities in your ED? Fact is, you can.

Interdependency (Interconnectedness) and Capacity to Serve

The components of any system (the servers) rarely work in isolation. A change to any one component often produces an effect somewhere else in the system. The servers are often affected by one another, particularly regarding their *availability for service.* This impacts the rates of resource utilization and patient throughput performance, and determines the overall *capacity of your ED to serve* as a total service system. It is very difficult to predict the effects that these interdependencies produce on system performance, including ED length of stay, particularly when, as is usually the case, significant variation is present at the same time.

Example: Variation and interdependency in a simple three-server system.

Patient Arrivals	Server 1	Server 2	Server 3
T: 10 min	T: 9 min	T: 9 min	T: 9 min

If patients arrive in this simple ED example at exactly 10-minute intervals and each stage of processing takes exactly 9 minutes, what is the average time a patient spends in this simple system? Because there is no variability in the system, the average time a patient spends in the department is 27 minutes. No waiting.

Now let us assume a more realistic scenario in that these are average times so that patients arrive on average every 10 minutes and it takes on average 9 minutes to serve a patient at each stage. What is the average time that a patient will spend in this system? This question is more difficult to answer because there is variability in both the patient arrival rates and the service processing times. We would expect that because things are not running as precisely as they did in the first example, waiting lines (queues) would begin to develop between each of the service stages. To confuse us further, the range of variability around the averages for arrivals and processing times are not given.

Most people would estimate that the average is still 27 minutes or maybe slightly longer, but this is not true. Assuming a typical range of variability (Robinson, 2004), the average time in the system is actually closer to 150 minutes! Yes.

So the compounding effects of variability and interdependency in a system make it very difficult to predict the overall performance of a system, even one as simple as this three-server model.

When ED managers and others try using averaged data to predict the service performance of their ED systems, those predictions are invariably wrong. However, both ED patients and the ED staff will certainly feel the effects of unreckoned variation and interdependency on the ED system, while patients wait in an overcrowded ED.

Complexity

With increasing *combinational* complexity (the number of components in a system or the number of combinations of system components available) and *dynamic* complexity (due to interactions of components over time) it becomes impossible to predict the performance of a system as actions are taken, staffing changes are made, and patient service loads (both demand and demand mix) vary, without some sophisticated science and new tools.

Simulation Modeling in the Emergency Department: All Patients Are Not the Same

Process simulation models are computer-generated graphic representations of dynamic systems under a variety of conditions.

Discrete event simulation (DES) modeling and software were designed, when computers hit the scene, to track "discrete events" as entities traveled through a queuing (service) system; that is, specific changes in state are tracked and time stamped as an entity moves through whatever queuing system is being modeled with the software. DES time clocks keep detailed track of all processing times and all waiting times, in the context of the arrival rates, which also vary over time. Through very complex mathematical analytic engines, DES models are able to explicitly represent variability, dependency, and interdependencies (= complexity) in a computer representation of any system.

Queuing systems consist of entities being processed through a series of service stages, with the opportunity for queues to form between each stage when there is insufficient processing capacity at server units, as in an ED.

Process simulations make it possible to predict how well an ED would perform under different conditions of volume, acuity, staff scheduling and staff mix, and so on. Computer models can be used to test resource deployment strategies (like staggering shifts or calling in additional help) or to determine the optimal mix of experienced nurses, physicians, and technicians that would be needed in the event of a terrorist bombing. A particularly useful application of computer modeling is in the design of new EDs.

You will need to have regular access to several types of performance metrics (operational data) to understand departmental *service performance*. The metrics that are particularly important to understanding the performance of any service system include resource utilization rates (how busy your nurses are compared to your docs or techs); where and when waiting (queuing) occurs; how various staffing (rostering) solutions affect throughput capacity and capacity to serve under various service loads (volume, acuity, and case mix). Accurate data is integral to informed decision making. Reliable ESI case mix data is a key metric for analyzing an ED's service performance. All patients are not the same.

Process Simulation Modeling and ESI Case Mix Data Summary

Process simulation modeling is useful for modeling queuing systems, that is, service systems. Queuing systems consist of customers being processed through a series of service stages, where there is the opportunity for queues (waiting lines) to form between stages when there is insufficient processing capacity at a server.

Queuing systems and the waiting problems associated with them are commonly found in health care settings. Health care facilities contain numerous examples of queuing systems and, not surprisingly, are often plagued by imbalances in demand and service capacity. Once ESI triage has been adopted and ESI presenting mix data is available, you could, with some help, use simulation modeling to answer questions about complex aspects of your ED's operations that are not otherwise analyzable. Process simulation modeling is essentially an approach to demand forecasting and capacity analysis decision making, quantitatively. It is a tool that allows one to evaluate demand and capacity matching solutions without disrupting ED operations. In fact, it was the potential to apply computer modeling in the complex ED setting that originally drove the development of ESI triage.

Anyone interested can obtain, at no cost, ESI triage, version 4, from www. ahrq.gov/research/esi. One can download a pdf version of the *Implementation Handbook*, fully licensed, directly from this site; or request that one free copy of the spiral-bound *Implementation Handbook* and *Everything You Need To Know* training DVD be mailed to you (Figure 1.3).

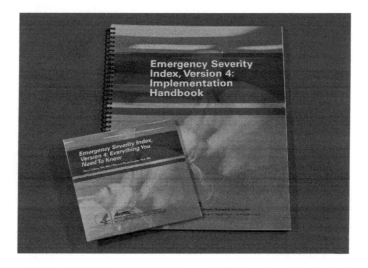

Figure 1.3

References

Robinson, S. *Simulation: The Practice of Model Development and Use*, Wiley, 2004.

Chapter 2

Process Mapping and Workflow Diagramming in Health Care

Sueanne McKniff

Process *improvement* without process knowledge … is futile.

–Sueanne McKniff

Process improvement attempts, in the absence of focused process investigation and accurate documentation, are frequently an effort in futility. Most health care workers can recount at least one tale of the phenomenon that occurs as a result of the efforts of well-intentioned employees who invest time, resources, and energy to remedy problems. These efforts repeatedly produce unpredictable and undesirable results, which become apparent as the downstream effects emerge. Initial improvements may be obtained, albeit the success is frequently transient and the results unsustainable.

Here's what happens: Imagine that someone baked a cake without a comprehensive list of ingredients and it turned out, well, let's say gross. They would then attempt to improve the cake by randomly increasing some ingredients while limiting or omitting others. This is the approach behind the process improvement that is frequently applied in the health care arena. Many of the processes in health care were never actually engineered; instead they just evolved, slowly, over time. As the complexity, acuity, and volume of the patients who are requesting health care resources continue to increase, meticulous attention to efficient system-wide throughput will be crucial to demand capacity matching.

The solution to process improvement lies in a quite basic concept: to improve the process you must understand the process. W. Edwards Deming summed it up nicely: "Every process is perfectly designed to produce exactly the results it produces."

Does performance improvement imply to "beat 'em with a larger stick" at your organization? *"Maybe it is the process causing the problem not the people."*

It is imperative to pursue a culture that focuses less on blaming the masses and more on simplifying and error proofing the broken processes in which staff are subjected to work. Imagine if staff members in an inpatient care unit reported every time they *almost* made an error or when reworks or a delay occurred while providing patient care. Future process failures could be prevented by process analysis and improvement. This, regrettably, is not the atmosphere throughout most health care organizations today, where the preliminary action often is to blame and reprimand. Reeducation for the staff member might be considered; however, this still implies fault on the part of the provider. When a patient codes in post-op, the first question is, Who was the nurse? A 29-year-old patient with chest pain evolves into an acute myocardial infarction while in the waiting room of an emergency department; the question again is, Who was the nurse?

There are no bad people, only bad processes.

—W. Edwards Deming

What Is a Process?

A process is a sequence of specific actions required to perform a task or series of tasks from the moment the activity begins until the tasks are completed. If we were in the business of making chocolate bonbons, the process and the delays would be tangible. Manufacturing environments have the advantage of being able to see the product throughout the production phases. In health care, the product is service delivery. Constant variability, as a result of provider preferences and the uniqueness of each individual patient, presents an increased challenge of process documentation. Process engineering tools have been employed by other service industries for decades, such as the airline industry, grocery stores, and even amusement parks.

The Institute for Health Care Improvement (2003) recognizes that "the answer to improving flow of patients lies in redesigning the overall, system-wide work processes that create the flow problems."

To fix any process, one must first understand how work flows through the processes, then eliminate unnecessary steps and focus on improving the flow. The key subprocesses and decision points within that system must be identified, and fix those that need to be fixed. Problems that persist may require a systems-level approach to resolve.

Health care improvement advisory groups are challenging health care institutions with recommendations and mandates directed at patient flow and workflow efficiency improvement efforts.

The leaders develop and implement plans to identify and mitigate impediments to efficient patient flow throughout the hospital.

—Joint Commission flow standard LD.3.15

The Institute of Medicine (IOM) introduced the six quality "aims": safe, timely, effective, efficient, equitable, and patient centered. Historically, health care administrators have been attempting to address the resulting problems, which unknowingly stemmed from flawed systems. Despite honest and driven attempts of quality improvement initiatives, efforts have been repetitively unsuccessful and this is attributed to the lack of process analysis. The processes and subprocesses within health care have rarely been evaluated; in fact, many were never actually designed to begin with; they simply evolved over time.

The education and subsequent application of engineering of manufacturing-derived methodologies that health care organizations are experiencing can have a positive impact through the application of some simple engineering tools.

"Seeing" a Process

It may seem ridiculous to mention how to "see" a process, but tasks that are familiar are thought of as one entity instead of being seen as the numerous and frequently complex activities required for process completion.

Imagine that every time you typed your name, you had to think of each individual letter. Instead, your brain thinks of your name and your fingers make it appear on the screen. When a complex process is taught to someone for the first time, it must be done in dissected steps. An example of this is when an experienced surgeon effortlessly slides a central line into a patient's chest. It is graceful and simple. To teach this procedure it must be broken down to a painful level of detail, such as when to open the gloves and even at which phase of the process the gloves should be donned. A substantial amount of work goes into listing the order of the activity steps, and crucial details will be omitted if the educational document is not created while directly observing the process.

An exciting event is when workflow diagrams are shown to stakeholders or frontline staff for the first time. It is illuminating for various reasons: robust discussions dictate process variation, provider preferences, policies, nonpolicies, and culture issues that dictate process flow ensue. While consensus regarding the steps of the process is the desired deliverable, the conversations are priceless in the pursuit of standardized work.

Workflow Analysis Is Relevant in the Absence of a Problem

Installation of an information system is an example of the use of workflow analysis in the absence of a problem. Identification of the current state of a process and the creation of workflow diagrams prior to the go-live date will improve the potential of successful installation and decrease the probability of automating bad processes. This discovery exercise will also identify interfaces to existing systems and documents, and allow for the accurate forecasting of a needs list for workstations, handheld devices, monitors, and the like.

There may be a need to negotiate a compromise between the current patient care delivery process and the information system prior to installation. Limitations of the system or the inability to support current processes will become evident if workflow analysis occurs prior to the installation. Here is an example: In the current patient care process the nurse documents on a patient prior to registration, but the process dictated by information systems (IS) is that there will not be anywhere for the nurse to document information until after some level of registration is complete.

A team of appropriate stakeholders and frontline staff members' involvement with the creation and validation of the workflow is an important part of a workflow analysis project. Creation of new diagrams that include proposed process changes post-IS installation are frequently referred to "future state" workflow diagrams. These diagrams may also serve as a communication tool depicting the impending process changes for frontline staff to be made aware. Consider naming the diagrams as "pre-go live" and "post-go live" because "current state" and "future state" become out of date the week of the IS installation.

Workflow Analysis for Problem Resolution

Formulate, in terms that are as specific as possible, the problem and forecast the desired process improvement deliverables. What you have identified as the problem is often the symptom(s) of a problem and not the actual problem. "Improving" a symptom may initially appear to alleviate the problem, but could actually make the problem worse.

Process efficiency problems usually stem from a process or a state of difficulty that negatively affects the delivery of patient-focused care. Stratification of each step within a process is necessary to reveal the handoffs, waiting episodes, and variation that may impede efficient patient-care delivery. The key is to initially focus on understanding the processes, not on finding solutions.

Workflow is the series of activity steps and decision points that occurs for an entire process to be completed. A flowchart is a tool used to visually describe these steps. Flowcharting provides a graphic, picturelike representation to record process information in an easily understandable format. The terms *workflow diagram*, *process diagram*, and *process map* all refer to the documentation of the process; terms such as *workflow analysis* and *process analysis* refer to the analytical phase of an improvement project.

Because most health care processes were not actually engineered, it is safe to say that most processes have never even been examined. The course of process exploration will be an eye opener and may, for the first time, provide an illuminating view of workflow. Flowcharting and subsequent analysis is the technique that provides the means to thoroughly understand the nature of a problem, a necessary basis for problem resolution. "When no one notices a problem, it is likely to persist and may even grow bigger. While it remains unnoticed it will still have a detrimental effect upon operations" (Wheeler, 1993, 53).

Before Creating a Flowchart, Some Things to Consider

- Consult with the research department to see if approval from the institutional review board (IRB) is needed for your project.
- Evaluate the project importance. Consult an executive in the organization to assist with an evaluation of strategic alignment (high risk, Joint Commission mandated, Blue Book contained).
- Align the timing of the project with other initiatives in any particular clinical environment.
- Include participants from all departments that have direct or indirect process involvement.
- Complete a project charter and obtain champion support.
- Complete a SIPOC (supplier, inputs, process, outputs, and customers) exercise to aid in the identification of correct project team members and scope of the project.
- Draft a scripted sentence to communicate to frontline staff the nature and purpose of the observation. This "elevator speech" will be repeated many times for many people, preferably without them having to ask why you are watching them. It should include something about a goal to make it easier for them to accomplish the work they are trying to do, to find flaws in the process, and to help them do their work easier. The use of a scripted sentence should decrease the extent of the Hawthorne effect.

About Observing the Process

Don't Rely on Memory of the Process

Go to the front line and observe the work where the work is being done. "Get your shoes dirty" with the frontline people. Workflow documents are frequently drafted in rooms with large posters or dry erase boards as teams are led through performance improvement exercises. The result of such an exercise cannot be a substitution for workplace observation; success lies heavily in the subsequent validation of the workflow diagrams by the frontline staff that actually does the work.

If the desired workflow diagram is of a proposed future state, certainly gather all information necessary from all stakeholders and draft a workflow diagram. But if the process identified is a current state process, you must observe it to document it correctly. If you expect to sit in your office and document processes exclusively from the perspective of your desk, close this book and go for coffee; it will be a better use of your time.

Who Should Observe the Process?

Be cognizant when the observation is done by managers, since frontline staff will be very suspicious that they are personally under observation instead of the process being scrutinized. Process owners may be too close to the process to objectively and correctly identify all activity steps and decision points; however, someone with no experience in the field may be unsuccessful at navigation of the work process. The luxury of additional staff with time allotted to assist with such projects is rare. Creative solutions have included filming the process (not an option in the health care arena because of confidentiality issues), and the use of college students, premed students, and medical students. The highest yield of success may be achieved, in teaching institutions, from residents who have a vested interest (i.e., a research project). Keep in mind that individuals with minimal clinical exposure will experience difficulty navigating the environment and have less of an ability to recognize documentation-worthy events. Whoever the observer, they should be prepared to deliver the scripted sentence to frontline staff to explain the purpose of the observation.

Keep Out of the Process

The intention is to observe and document the process while avoiding the temptation to permeate the process. For example, a resident observing the intake of patients with chest pains in a busy emergency department; the triage nurse was unable to resist the convenience of consulting the resident for advanced triage orders (CT scans, etc.).

Who Should be Observed?

To capture the variation in the process it is important to observe a variety of staff and work times: new staff as well as senior staff, busy times in addition to slow. Do not dismiss the travelers (agency staff); and most important, remember night shift and weekend staff—they frequently function with their own set of rules.

Be sensitive that the current process was most likely developed by people still working in the organization. They and others may have emotional ties to the current process, aka "The way we've always done it."

Level of Detail

Depending on the complexity of the problem and the goal specified in the project charter, a high level of detail may be adequate. Document only the appropriate level of detail that is necessary to achieve the project goal. For example, it may suffice to have one activity step that states [page consultant]; however, if the scope of the problem encompasses the delay in getting a consultant to the bedside, then multiple steps would be indicated [present chart (*to unit clerk*)] → wait → receive chart (*unit clerk*) → read order → research telephone number, etc. Attempt to maintain a consistent level of detail throughout the workflow diagram.

What are We Looking For?

Remember that *you don't know what you don't know* about the process. There may be intradepartmental handoffs or some archaic paper process still in use simply because no one thought to stop doing it. Here are some thoughts to consider:

- Activity steps
- Sequence of the activity steps
- Decision points
- Handoffs (of any kind, inter- or intradepartmentally)
- Rework (multiple overhead phone pages because previous pages are not heard)
- Variation (not just provider-to-provider variation, but the same person will vary their execution of the process without cause)
- Waiting (not actual times, just the activity of waiting)
- Waste in extra steps. If multiple physical steps are necessary for process completion, reflect the concern in the wording of the activity step. If this movement appears to be a substantial time constraint in the process resulting from the location of equipment or supplies, a spaghetti diagram would be an additional tool to document the waste in motion.

Silos

Silos are departments or groups working in isolation from one another. A process that relies on the resources or actions of another department for process completion must be involved in the workflow diagramming process. For example, if workflow diagrams need to be created in preparation for a medication distribution of a documentation system install, it is not appropriate for the pharmacy to independently complete its workflow and the inpatient nurses to complete theirs. It is the interface between the two departments where the greatest potential for process error exists.

Make 'em Ugly

Create a diagram that provides an accurate reproduction of workflow; don't be afraid to make it "ugly" by showing all of the unnecessary steps in the current processes. Reveal the places where variation, delay, rework, redundancy, and interdependency affect the typical work process. These diagrams are not created for the Joint Commission or for teaching the process to new employees; they are created to find the ugly, broken portions of the process that make it virtually impossible for staff to function efficiently or effectively.

How to Capture the Initial Observations

You will need to choose an initial method in which to quickly jot a few notes while you are observing in the workplace. It must allow you to function quickly and portably. It might be a tablet PC, a legal tablet with a pencil, or sticky notes and a clipboard. Creating preliminary notes in outline form is easily understood and logical to most people, but the speed and flexibility achieved with the sticky notes technique are tremendous.

Outline technique: The outline technique is simply that—an outline (or a list) of the activity steps and decision points of the process. Create a list or use bullet points, but do not number the activities; the sequencing will change or additional steps will be added during subsequent observations. If using a paper tablet, consider skipping a few lines between activities for the addition of later entries. List the activity steps in any kind of sentence structure that comes to mind. Note: A consistent format of noun first, followed by a verb should be used when the final diagrams are created.

Pro: Does not require the adoption of any new skills or special materials.

Con: It is harder to alter the order or to insert additional activity steps between the sentences. The nature of an outline format makes it appear that data is complete. Decision points and handoffs are not visibly evident.

The information must now be transferred from the outline to sticky notes or a computer flowcharting graphics program. Capturing the decision points and handoffs will illuminate variability and generate process questions to be answered during subsequent observations. With experience and practice, the workflow diagram could be created directly onto a computer graphics program.

Sticky Notes Technique

Each activity step or decision point is written directly onto a sticky note. Any size sticky note will do, but the rectangular 1.5 × 2 inch size is perfect. Place the note directly onto a legal tablet while observing the process. Inevitably, after a sticky note is placed, it will become apparent that a previous step was skipped. Simply move the sticky notes into the correct order. The sticky notes come in various colors. The different colors can be used to identify process details such as the role of who is acting on that activity step or to identify an activity by another department. List the activity steps in any kind of sentence structure that comes to mind. Note: A consistent format of noun first, followed by a verb will be used when the final diagrams are created.

Pro: Increased ease of seeing the process and reorganizing the order of the activity steps as they are discovered. It also is very easy to visualize the difference between activity steps and decision points. Staff members, in addition to the scribe, are quickly able to see the flow of formation and can easily redirect the flow capture as well as add additional information. This approach to data gathering allows for a great amount of process understanding to happen prior to attempting to create the workflow diagram in a software tool.

Con: This is a foreign concept and initially creates the appearance of being disorganized. However, because the process may exhibit a high level of disarray this technique lends itself to the task quite nicely.

Transfer to an Electronic Document

Which type of flowchart is best?

a. Standard flowchart diagram (a single linear flow diagram) (Figure 2.1): The standard flowchart is intuitively easy to understand and easy to create. The process flows from the top of the page to the bottom. It is best for small processes or ones with minimal handoffs.

b. Cross-functional diagram (swim lanes) (Figure 2.2): Initially, the cross-functional diagram is more complex to understand. "Swim lanes" clarify the provider/department role in the process being evaluated, in a quick and easy to locate manner. An information lane provides an easy solution to identify the information resources necessary to accomplish each activity. Cross-functional diagrams may be more time intensive to master.

   Note: The numbers associated with some of the activity steps identify the portions of the process which a time data study through direct observation could be conducted.

Flow Chart Symbols (See Figure 2.3)

Your organization may have additional standards for workflow diagramming; contact IS, project management, or your quality department. There may be prepared templates, educational tutorials, or even mentors or resources that may be able to assist with to the project.

Standardized symbols exist to improve consistency in flowchart creation:

- ◾ **Ovals** represent the start and end points of the process.
  - There may be multiple end points to one start point.
- ◾ **Squares** represent one step/activity.
  - Use verb–noun labeling (e.g., *complete triage* or *obtain cultures*).
  - Clarify role in parentheses and italicize. Not necessary for cross-functional (swim lane) diagrams.
- ◾ **Diamonds** represent decision points.
  - Each decision point usually has only two exit points.
  - Phrase the decision questions to yield either a yes or no answer, or two distinct possibilities. Determine acuity. From the diamond would be two flows, one labeled "high acuity" and the other "low acuity."
- ◾ **On and off-page references** link the activity steps when more than one page is required. Connectors is the fifth symbol. If the process must repeat a sequence of activity steps, the entire sequence can either be rewritten or use a connector line to reenter the process above that series of activity steps.

Including Personal Names

Personal names are only appropriate in the document if found to be extremely useful in explaining the process to end users during the creation and validation phase [e.g., present chart (*to Melody*)]. However, because this will serve as a historical document and most likely be used for other projects and by other departments within the organization, it is preferable to substitute personal names with job titles [i.e., present chart (*to chart reviewer*)]. If the person or the discipline is important to specify, consider transferring the information into a cross-functional diagram.

Color Coding Activity Steps

When creating a standard flowchart it is difficult to quickly identify a series of activity steps for a particular role or department. Coloring each set of activity steps in a different color is helpful for this purpose. Again, consider the benefits of transferring the data to a cross-functional diagram.

Color Coding "Off-Page" References

If the workflow encompasses multiple pages, on-page and off-page reference shapes electronically link the diagram. If printing the diagrams is necessary, as when sharing with stakeholders, the linking of the software is lost. It is useful to label the references as to the page where the workflow goes to or comes from. One workflow depicting an organization's revenue stream spanned 22 pages; the interdependency and reworks in the process necessitated multiple on/off references on each page. Each set of references was given a color to quickly navigate through the complex process while on paper, which, as you might imagine, was taped to the administrative director's wall for quick reference during the project.

Date the Documents

When saving the documents electronically, date them and keep copies for version control; consider using a share point sight. Select one person to be the workflow diagram architect for consistency in documentation style.

Watch for Scope Creep

Remember to refer to the project charter to evaluate for scope creep. Scope creep is the desire to collect data or become distracted by issues that fall outside of the boundaries of the project and the original problem/goal statements. Stay within the scope of the project to increase your likelihood of a quick success. Create an organized list "parking lot" of these additional issues/problems for future exploration.

Work Sessions and Interactive Meetings

Workflow diagrams provide a perfect platform for workgroup meetings. Projection of the diagrams on a screen or wall enables large groups to focus on a particular area of the process. Use a square (vs. a rectangle, and larger than an activity step) and color the square to document questions or action steps determined by the work group. Consider making a ledger on the first or last page to indicate the date of the notes/action steps/questions depicted in the "red squares."

Validate the Diagrams

The process has been observed, documented, revised, and reviewed with a few subject matter experts, and then revised again. For some projects it would be appropriate to begin to analyze the diagrams. However, if the purpose is a substantial project, conduct formal workflow validation sessions. Organize these validation sessions and invite a predetermined number of frontline staff (perhaps two staff members from each department, disciplines, experience levels, and shifts). Explain that the diagrams are merely a draft to serve as a platform for discussion and brainstorming.

Revisions to the documents will most likely be necessary and possibly time consuming. This should be taken into account when creating the project management timeline.

Discussion

At a time when health care is in such crisis, it may be tempting to transfer "best practices" from similar institutions to your organization. Evaluating the best practices may be informative, albeit, it is imperative to understand your organization's specific workflows laden with ugly processes and culture issues. These are the process issues which, when reengineered, will produce high yielding sustainable results.

Don't underestimate the importance of collaboration with frontline staff from all involved departments during the workflow exploration, documentation and validation phases. Creating workflows together and learning to see the same process in different ways identifies different opinions of the same workflow process. Implementation of the improved process will be adopted more readily when those most affected by the change—the process owners—are the champions of the change initiative.

It will be beneficial to remind the project team not to randomly make isolated "improvements" as process issues are illuminated. Wait for the "as-is" workflow to be captured, then craft the proposed future state processes to provide tailored results. It is dangerous to alter one portion of a process without consideration for the process as a whole. Unpredicted undesirable downstream effects will result.

Conclusion

Many of today's health care service delivery units are large, complex environments marred with scars from failed "performance" rather than process improvement attempts. Personality traits exhibited by the practitioners who have been surviving in these circumstances are conditioned to and demanding of immediate gratification from quick fixes, and are used to working around the inefficiencies in the process. The time consumption required by careful process identification, analysis, and data collection could reinforce the practitioner's belief that administration is unaware of the current problematic state. Careful education and involvement of staff prior to the execution phase is imperative to the buy-in of staff and successful long-term process excellence.

The approach of randomly making changes and hoping to improve processes wastes time and resources. The application of a few simple tools using process evaluation methodologies will not. Knowing the amount of time required for each step of the process and the resources necessary for each step will be useful to operational decision making. Initial consistency in problem identification through process identification, process analysis, and activity/process standardization will increase group cohesiveness, a feeling of success, and the efficiency of subsequent process improvement projects.

References

Andersen, B., and Fagerhaug, T. *Root Cause Analysis: Simplified Tools and Techniques.* Milwaukee, WI: ASQ Quality Press, 2000.

Bossidy, L., and Charan, R. *Execution: The Discipline of Getting Things Done.* New York: Crown Business, 2002.

Bowen, H.K. "Designing Caregiver- and Patient-Centered Health Care Systems." In *Building a Better Delivery System: A New Engineering/Health Care Partnership,* edited by P. Reid, D. Compton, J. Grossman, and G. Fanjiang, 135–140. Washington, DC: National Academies Press, 2005.

Brassard, M., and Ritter, D. *Sailing through Six Sigma: How the Power of People Can Perfect Processes and Drive Down Costs.* Concord, NH: Capital Offset Company, 2002.

Caldwell, C., Brexler, J., and Gillem, T. *Lean-Six Sigma for Healthcare: A Senior Leader Guide to Improving Cost and Throughput.* Milwaukee, WI: ASQ Quality Press, 2005.

George, M.L. *Lean Six Sigma for Service.* New York: McGraw-Hill, 2003.

George, M.L. *Lean Six Sigma Pocket Tool Book.* New York: McGraw-Hill, 2005.

Institute for Healthcare Improvement (IHI). *Optimizing Patient Flow: Moving Patients Smoothly through Acute Care Settings.* IHI Innovation Series white paper. Boston: Institute for Healthcare Improvement, 2003.

Institute of Medicine (IOM). *To Err Is Human: Building a Safer Health System.* Washington, DC: National Academies Press, 2000.

Institute of Medicine (IOM). *Crossing the Quality Chasm: A New Health System for the 21st Century.* Washington, DC: National Academies Press, 2001.

Joint Commission on Accreditation of Healthcare Organizations (JCAHO). *2005 Comprehensive Accreditation Manual for Hospitals: The Official Handbook (CAMH).* Oak Brook, IL: Joint Commission Resources, 2005.

Peach, R.W. *The Memory Jogger 9000/2000: A Pocket Guide to Implementing the ISO 9001 Quality Systems Standard.* Salem NH: Goal/QPC, 2000.

Quest Worldwide Consulting. *The Lean Toolbox: Tools for Lean Operating.* Quest Worldwide Education, 1999.

Reid, P., Compton, D., Grossman, J., and Fanjiang, G. *Building a Better Delivery System: A New Engineering/Health Care Partnership.* Washington, DC: National Academies Press, 2005.

Walton, M. *The Deming Management Method.* New York: Berkley Publishing Group, 1986.

Wheeler, D.J. *Understanding Variation: The Key to Managing Chaos.* Knoxville, TN: SPC Press, 1993.

Womack, J., and Jones, D.T. *Lean Thinking: Banish Waste and Create Wealth in Your Corporation.* New York: Simon & Schuster, 1996.

Womack, J., Jones, D.T., and Roos, D. *The Machine That Changed the World.* New York: Simon & Schuster, 1990.

Chapter 3

What is Lean Six Sigma?
An Introduction to Lean and Six Sigma for the Health Care Novice

David Eitel

Why Lean?

Lean is a highly effective business improvement methodology that is commonly used in manufacturing. These principles applied to the services delivery side of decision making have the potential to dramatically improve both the efficiency and quality of hospital and health system care delivery systems, while lowering costs and improving staff morale.

"But we don't make cars" many health care professionals would say. However, these methods and its associated tools (with only minor occasional differences) apply to services delivery just as well as manufacturing, including health care. At the ED Lead with Lean training sessions two winters ago, Doug Sears highlighted the following:

Goals of the Lean Business Improvement Method: Making better business decisions
1. With intimate knowledge about the customer
2. With intimate knowledge about the process
3. With data
4. With the right people involved

What really irks me is that investment analysts always talk about ITT's Value-Based Lean Six Sigma effort, or others like it, as cost reduction. It's not cost reduction. If you're doing cost reduction you're taking out people, you're skimping here, you're cutting back on an investment there: that's cost reduction. This is process change. Yes, you might take out resources, whether they be capacity, dollars, people, material, whatever it is, but it's not because you're cutting them, you don't need them; you've found a better way to get the work done.

—Lou Giuliano, CEO of ITT

What Is Lean?

The Lean principles of business management come to us from Toyota. They derive from Taiichi Ohno's Toyota Production Methods that he evolved over 30 years. (Ohno never used the term *Lean*. Womack et al. [1991] coined the term in their book *The Machine That Changed the World*.) Lean in manufacturing is all about a rigorous analysis of demand, then working to create a "single piece flow" approach to delivering products to customers.

Word Associations

The following are some common word associations that come to mind to audiences when they are given the name "Toyota":

1. Reliable
2. Well designed
3. Affordable
4. Great gas mileage (efficient)

What if a couple of years from now, patients who came into any care delivery setting said the same things about their experience when they left? (Well, maybe not the gas mileage comment.)

Lean Principles

Lean is also often called process excellence. Lean principles analyze processes to *maximize process velocity* (i.e., velocity of the entity going through the process) *and quality* by reducing wasteful utilization of resources and reducing complexity. We offer four elevator speeches regarding Lean for your consideration:

Elevator Speech #1: Lean is about achieving service process excellence by getting rid of waste.

Elevator Speech #2: Lean is about flowing patients through the business unit/ system under discussion.

Lean principles improve speed through the process without reducing quality by *reducing nonvalue added activities from the work.* Lean principles distinguish between productive (meaningful) work and those activities that increase cost without contributing any benefit to the customer, like waiting (= waste).

Elevator Speech #3: Lean principles allow for the visualization of cost reduction opportunities where they were never before seen, with very little outlay of capital.

Elevator Speech #4: Lean principles leverage the return on invested capital, which, in services like health care, to a large extent is due to human resources.

In Lean, decision making is supported by data. The core data in a Lean business improvement initiative are derived from process maps. All Lean tools require the use of data, derived from workflow analysis, to guide decision making.

Six Sigma

Healthcare is the only industry I have ever heard of that actually has a name for a major category of waste. You have waiting rooms. Most organizations outside of health care would go bankrupt if they thought like this.

—Quality expert (as quoted in Caldwell et al. 2005, 33)

The Six Sigma methods of business management come to us from Motorola of Japan. With Six Sigma, one goes after specific opportunities to *eliminate defects* to improve quality and *reduce costs in major ways.* Six Sigma uses some highly quantitative, advanced statistical methods, and therefore often uses Master Black Belts and Black Belts to help to plan and manage projects, and Green Belts to help get them done. Six Sigma requires a major institutional commitment and a cultural change to be effective.

What Is a Sigma?

See Figure 3.1.

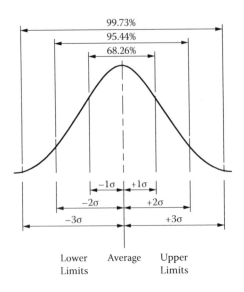

Sigma = a Standard Deviation
A Greek letter that represents the variation around the average (i.e., one standard deviation)
<u>Six</u> Sigma means that only 3.4 defects happen per million opportunities to make the error
The greater the sigma, the smaller the variation = the fewer the errors (defects)

Figure 3.1

Defects Per Million Opportunities: DPMO Thinking Applied to Health Care

Unfortunately, unlike manufacturing, healthcare has no traditional quality measures based on "per million" anything. We simply do not produce a million medications or a million cardiac surgeries. Healthcare measures quality almost universally as a percentage (nosocomial infection rates, mortality rate, x-ray re-take rate, etc.). In healthcare the DPMO concept confuses nurses, physicians and other staff and adds no value to the measurement of quality. Rather, it is best to convert the DPMO concept to a "per hundred" or percentage, which is easily understood by physicians, nurses, and others. DPMO is simply "per million" with 6 zeroes; a percentage can be derived by moving the decimal four places to the left. For example, 3-sigma is 66,000 DPMO; to convert to a percentage, simply move the decimal four places to the left to produce 6.6%. All staff members understand 6.6%; none understand 66,000 DPMO.

—Caldwell et al. (2005, 157)

Table 3.1 is Caldwell et al.'s (2005) summary of DPMO from the book *Lean-Six Sigma for Healthcare*. Represented are sigma levels; then the associated DPMO number of occurrences (i.e., defect [error] rate occurrence); error rate converted to a percent; quality yield, which is the rate in percent that no errors therefore occur; then the estimation of the associated cost of poor quality as a percent of any business unit/system's total operating costs.

If you think this to be approximately correct, what percent of your service unit's total operating budget is consumed by the cost of poor quality, right now?

Table 3.1

Sigma Level	DPMO	Error as a Percent	Quality Yield	Cost of Quality/Cost of Poor Quality as Percent of Total Operating Costs
2	308,537	30.8 = 31%	69%	Uncompetitive
3	66,807	6.7%	93.3%	25%–40%
4	6,219	.6%	99.4%	15%–25%
5	233	.0233%	99.98%	5%–15%
6	3.4	.00034%	99.9997%	World class

Source: Reproduced with permission from C. Caldwell, J. Brexler, and T. Gillem, *Lean Six-Sigma for Healthcare: A Senior Leader Guide to Improving Cost and Throughput* (Milwaukee, WI: ASQ Quality Press, 2005).

DMAIIC (pronounced de-MAY-ic) is the acronym used to describe the mandatory steps required of this very disciplined Six Sigma business process performance improvement method:

Design
Measure
Analyze
Improve
Implement
Control

Acknowledgment

I acknowledge the former YH ED Health Services Design Team.

References

Caldwell, C., Brexler, J., and Gillem, T. 2005. *Lean Six-Sigma for Healthcare: A Senior Leader Guide to Improving Cost and Throughput*. Milwaukee, WI: ASQ Quality Press.
Womack, J.P., Jones, D.T., and Roos, D. 1991. *The Machine That Changed the World*. New York: HarperPerennial.

Chapter 4

Using Lean Six Sigma to Accelerate Emergency Department Results

Greg Butler, Chip Caldwell, and Shannon Elswick

The team that makes the fewest mistakes wins.

**—Assistant Football Coach Chan Caldwell,
University of Tennessee, 1946–1954**

Quality systems, like Lean Six Sigma, by definition are change models, intended to stimulate creativity and mold the environment for change within the organization. When applied systemically in a standardized, disciplined manner, quality systems add the important element of learning loops, thereby enabling managers within the organization to learn from their collective successes and failures. All too often, health care senior leaders, unlike their manufacturing senior leader counterparts, fail to recognize that a quality system is an organization-wide change model, as opposed to simply Joint Commission compliance or patient safety or other delegable objectives, and, thereby, fail to benefit from the power of quality constructs like Lean, Six Sigma, and the Toyota Production System.

However, many senior leaders in health care have recognized, either through wisdom or intuition, that as the degree of involvement of senior leaders in driving the effectiveness of the change model increases the magnitude of strategic results increases.

The purpose of this chapter is to highlight the importance of the following:

■ The role of senior leaders in optimizing the effectiveness of the use of Lean Six Sigma in an organization

■ The nondelegable roles of senior leaders versus the ineffectiveness of delegating the change model to individual department managers

■ Approaching improvement imperatives from a senior leader-driven "Big Quality" (Big Q) strategy deployment of sequences of projects over time versus a "little quality" (little q) one-project-at-a-time approach

■ The critical importance of the accountability structure versus a belief that Lean Six Sigma alone will produce sustainable results

■ The use of quality systems as organization-wide change models, and Lean Six Sigma in particular, can accelerate and assure sustainability of an organization's emergency department (ED) improvement efforts

Cases in Point

One of the major missteps made by executive leaders in Lean Six Sigma deployments is to behave as if Lean Six Sigma is simply a project methodology. In many instances this is the fault of consultants who may be exceptional Black Belts but who have never served in a senior leadership capacity in health care and lead executive teams down the path of selecting projects at the department manager accountability level versus at the vice president accountability level. This misstep is the kiss of death for any Lean Six Sigma initiative. Executives may play a passive, oversight role for a few months, perhaps even a year, but sooner or later executives will begin to skip steering committee meetings, engage in side talk, or leave early. This occurs not because executives do not value their own contributions, but rather because executives begin to realize that project selection by committee is not a role that can remain top of mind for an effective executive. However, as Dr. Joseph Juran observed, "Results happen one project at a time and in no other way" (Caldwell et al. 2009). Therefore, to effectively maintain the Lean Six Sigma infrastructure, executives need to have some sense of the potential impact of Lean Six Sigma project methods. The following case studies provide some sense of the nondelegable roles of senior leaders, the change model infrastructure, and results potential of a Lean Six Sigma strategic application. As the cases unfold, look for hints with an explanation in parentheses suggesting evidence of key success factors that will be reviewed in the section following the case study presentations.

Morton Plant Medical Center, Clearwater, Florida

During routine management oversight activities, Phil Beauchamp, CEO of Morton Plant Hospital in Clearwater, Florida, reviewed emergency department performance indicators with Lisa Johnson, vice president of patient services, and a Lean Six Sigma consultant (Caldwell et al. 2009). Although ED patient satisfaction was near the national average, at Morton Plant *average* is not in the management glossary. At that moment, Beauchamp committed himself and all the resources that might be required to help the ED leadership move from average to world-class performance.

> About Morton Plant Hospital
> - 687-bed tertiary-care center, level II ED
> - 55,744 ED visits annually
> - First U.S. hospital to win all categories of Top 100
> - Sterling Quality Award (Baldrige-based)
> Sources: Morton Plant Hospital (2008) and Caldwell et al. (2009).

Having won the prestigious Florida Sterling Quality Award and becoming one of the first U.S. hospitals to be recognized in all categories of the *Top 100*® lists, the executive team and middle management at Morton Plant possess a passion to be recognized in their community and around the nation for providing high-quality care while minimizing waste due to poor quality. Adopting Lean Six Sigma as a key deployment methodology in the ED to achieve its goal of becoming world class, Morton Plant took another step in its quality evolution.

Upon adopting the 100-Day Workout approach (key success factor: accountability structure) and the accelerating concepts of Lean Six Sigma, the Morton Plant ED achieved a 26-percent improvement in length of stay (LOS), as shown in Figure 4.1. The "exhaust" of this process improvement raised ED patient satisfaction scores from the 61st percentile to above the 90th percentile, while recovering over $4 million in bottom-line cost recovery.

St. Vincent's Medical Center, Jacksonville, Florida

CEO Scott Whalen, PhD, drew chuckles as he opened St. Vincent's Medical Center's third 100-Day Workout Summation, observing, "Variation is evil" (Ford 2007). As illustrated in Figure 4.2, during the next 2 hours five subteam leaders, representing the contiguous subprocesses that make up the ED–Inpatient

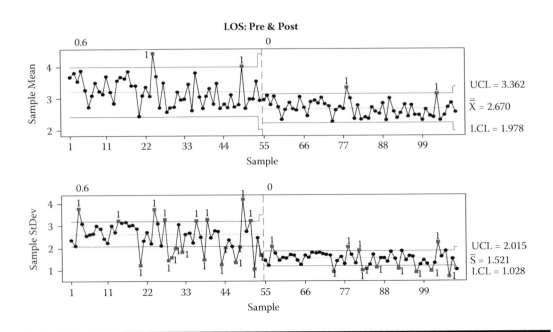

Figure 4.1   Morton Plant ED LOS improved 26 percent (Caldwell et al. 2009).

Bed Management care continuum, presented the results of their efforts during this 100-Day Workout. (Key success factor: Big Quality factor of organizing two or more subprocess teams working simultaneously on a large core process versus one small subprocess team working alone.)

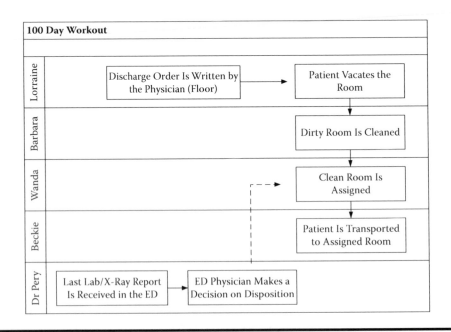

Figure 4.2   St. Vincent's 100-Day Workout organizational structure. (Reproduced with permission from Chip Caldwell & Associates, LLC, files.)

About St. Vincent's Medical Center
  – 528-bed teaching hospital
  – Owned by St. Vincent Health System
  – Affiliated with Ascension Health
  – HealthGrades "Distinguished Hospital"
Source: St. Vincent's Medical Center (2008).

As a result of multiple improvements by each of the subteams during each sequential 100-Day Workout cycle, St. Vincent's was able to achieve a 22-percent improvement in inpatient discharge time of day, thereby significantly reducing a major source of needless ED LOS-ED holds for inpatient beds as shown in Table 4.1. (Key success factor: Big Quality strategy deployment versus little quality one project at a time.)

The "exhaust" of this substantial removal of an ED bottleneck resulted in a 57-percent reduction in patients leaving the ED in a left-without-being-seen (LWBS) status, producing a bottom-line cost recovery of over $7 million (Caldwell and Butler 2009).

Table 4.1   Percent Discharges before 2 p.m.

Unit	Baseline	Summation
2E	46%	48%
2W	40%	53%
3E	44%	47%
3C	20%	52%
3W	29%	44%
4E	27%	36%
4C	37%	46%
4W	43%	57%
5E	51%	42%
5C	42%	47%
5W	27%	47%
5N	42%	54%
All	**37%**	**45%**
22% Improvement		

Source: Ford (2007, 7).

Dr. P. Phillips Hospital, Orlando, Florida

As she was discussing with the hospital president a project to evaluate and reduce patients who left the ED without treatment, Master Black Belt Debbie Goodwin said, "Lean Six Sigma always raises the bar. Depending upon where that bar is relative to the threshold, you're either trying to pull air from an empty dive tank or you're already back in the boat safely enjoying a refreshing drink." As a fellow diver and former high jumper, Shannon Elswick, FACHE, understood her analogy and encouraged her to be consistently aggressive when setting the bar.

About Dr. P. Phillips Hospital
- 237-bed community hospital
- Owned by Orlando Health
- 2008 Ivy Award Nominee for Hospitality by *Restaurants & Institutions* magazine
- Approximately 90,000 ED visits per year
- 30% of patients nonresident tourists/visitors and international travelers

The obvious challenge in an extremely high-volume ED like the one at Dr. P. Phillips Hospital (DPH) is to manage the ED throughput of this disproportionately high volume efficiently. Failure to do so results in patients who leave without treatment (LWT), leading to lost revenue and lost market share opportunity. During its first 100-Day Workout, the team at DPH identified several significant opportunities to positively impact this critical statistic.

The first breakthrough came from the immediate initiation and use of standardized clinical guidelines, especially those related to specimen collection. As Figure 4.3 and Figure 4.4 show, rapid cycle testing and subsequent changes in ancillary procedures demonstrated significantly positive results.

A significant process review of the actual triage flow led to the creation of a parallel (vs. serial) process for triage registration and a concurrent registration procedure. Staff members were redeployed and the triage area was physically restructured. The 100-Day Workout resulted in a 44-percent decrease in LWTs (with potential net revenue for each avoided LWT of approximately $448; Figure 4.5).

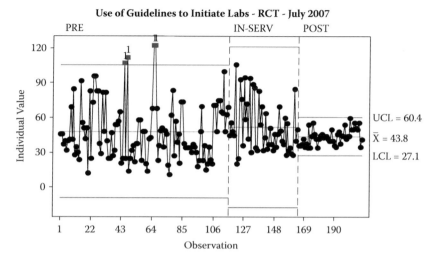

Figure 4.3 **ED left without treatment results.**

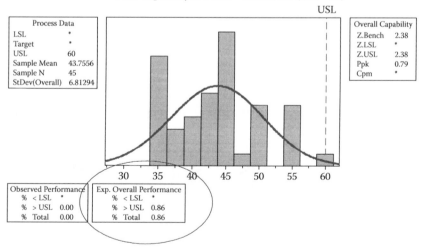

Figure 4.4 **100-Day Workout implementation structure. (Reproduced with permission from Caldwell et al., 2009.)**

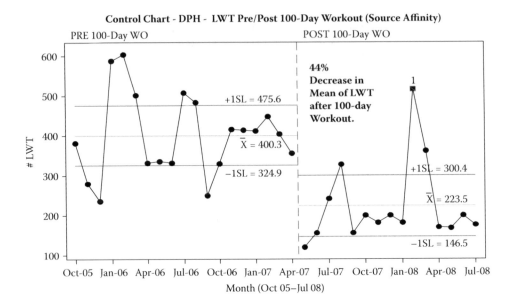

Figure 4.5   ED left without treatment results.

How Did They Get There? The Elements of an Effective Quality System

The answer to the question of how these distinguished organizations exceeded top quartile improvement is not simple, but it has a simple form. To achieve top quartile results, they mastered the following driving elements:

■ Big Quality strategic approach (versus little quality project mindset)
■ Accountability structure
■ Use of accelerating quality concepts like Lean Six Sigma

These three elements are discussed in detail next.

Big Quality Strategic Approach (versus Little Quality Project Mindset)

Many organizations approach the use of Lean Six Sigma or the Toyota Production System under the belief that the effective use of these accelerating quality concepts begins by training department-level managers and allocating resources to them. This, in our research, is not an effective route to achieving strategy-level results, often leaving senior leaders and board members disillusioned as to the effectiveness of these methods in health care. They fail to recognize that a one-project-at-at-time approach is a little q application. This approach often results because senior leaders believe they can simply delegate the use of these methods to Black Belts, none of whom have ever held senior leader roles, and, therefore, are set up for failure before they even begin.

Senior leaders responsible for quantum improvement recognize that the achievement of strategic-level results cannot be achieved via a one-project-at-a-time approach and certainly that the important roles of senior leaders cannot be delegated to Black Belts. Instead, senior leaders embrace their roles as follows (Butler and Caldwell 2008):

■ Set a three-year Big Q goal encompassing the entire ED continuum of care from ED patient presentation through the ED care process through bed management, ED nurse–floor nurse handoff, and transportation, until the patient was transported to the inpatient bed (for admitted patients).

■ Create a three-year project plan to achieve the Big Q goal that lays out a logical sequence of projects that will achieve the Big Q goal.

■ Assign a senior leader to be accountable for the result versus a passive, "come see me if you need me" role.

■ Assure that the critical components of the accountability structure are effectively performed. The management of the accountability structure is a non-delegable task of senior leaders but is often confused with the concepts contained within Lean Six Sigma. Senior leaders often assume that the Lean Six Sigma process, known as DMAIC (define, measure, analyze, improve, control), is all that is necessary to achieve a successful outcome and, thereby, mistakenly leave it up to the Black Belts to manage both the utilization of Lean Six Sigma concepts and the accompanying accountable structure for implementation. Top performing senior leaders separate the role of implementation as their key role, leaving the use of Lean Six Sigma concepts to those experts known as Black Belts. The elements of an effective accountable structure are discussed in detail in the section on the accountability structure.

■ Charter an ED physician team and a hospitalist team, setting the expectation that the physician practice change process was as important as other care and support processes.

Big Q Goal-Setting Process

In the authors' study "Secrets of Great Healthcare Organizations," an analysis of over two hundred U.S. hospitals, the goal-setting process was one of several differentiating characteristics separating top quartile performers from bottom quartile performers (Butler and Caldwell 2008; Pieper 2004). In top quartile performing organizations, the CEO and COO collaborate with the vice president who is accountable to the CEO and board for strategy achievement, becoming intimately involved in establishing the three-year stretch goal. Capitalizing on the power of Lean Six Sigma thinking as a strategic tool, Morton Plant and St. Vincent's senior leaders recognized that the ED is a critical entry point for admissions to the hospital and as a driver of the hospital's reputation in the community. Their designation of the ED as a "front door" to the organization distinguished the department as strategically important. By comparison, in bottom-quartile-performing organizations the goal-setting process is either little q, fail to involve the CEO, COO, and accountable vice president, or both, leaving the Black Belt to lay out the goal.

Moreover, senior leaders in top performing organizations recognize that Big Q core processes like the ED are not stand-alone functional departments, but rather are dependent upon the seamlessness of a host of to-follow processes like bed management, ED nurse–inpatient nurse communications, hospitalists' rounding patterns, transportation, and so forth. Therefore, to achieve a Big Q ED LOS, the change structure requires that representatives of these continuum functions enact improvements to their processes in tandem with ED subprocesses. Each participating subprocess team should be assigned a performance goal that, if achieved, would have a direct (preferably statistical) impact on ED LOS.

Another characteristic of top quartile performers is the ability to prioritize the critical from the noncritical. This important performance variable was reported by Jim Collins (2001) in his landmark study *Good to Great*. Prioritization is necessary to keep management's attention from being diluted beyond reasonable control. Executives, even with good intentions, have the tendency to simply put too much on their collective plates, with the result being poor execution and follow-through. Consequently, they are unable to accomplish some of their critical goals. This pitfall can be avoided by identifying core business processes that yield high leverage strategic results. Core care and business processes in most hospitals include:

- ED–inpatient bed management continuum
- Operations cost of quality (beyond productivity benchmarking, focusing on "in-quality staffing" and process waste)
- Surgical services (Big Q surgery beginning with case scheduling, through the pre-, peri-, and post-op processes, until the patient is in her/his inpatient bed or discharged)
- Patient care throughput (discharge time-of-day profile and number of minutes until the next patient is occupying the inpatient bed; most organizations approach patient care throughput with a little q mentality and, therefore, become frustrated that their discharge profiles fail to improve, even after the application of Lean Six Sigma)
- Intake services (physician offices, home health, some outpatient functions, and others that feed into acute care core processes)
- Care management/clinical decision making (length of stay and clinical utilization)
- Revenue cycle

A three-year strategic stretch goal can be determined for each of these core processes. Ownership of the goal must be assigned to an accountable vice president to deploy resources as needed to achieve the goal.

Setting Goals Using a Six Sigma Approach

Using Lean Six Sigma logic, both Morton Plant and St. Vincent's came to recognize that setting a benchmark for average LOS was not a productive exercise. Setting goals around average performance is a bit like stating, "I have one foot in hot water and the other in ice water, but on average I feel pretty comfortable." They applied this understanding and defined their goals in terms of the maximum acceptable LOS. In Lean Six Sigma terminology, this quality threshold is referred to as the upper specification limit (USL), that point beyond which LOS should not exceed. What USL actually represents is the voice of the customer. In other words, rather than focus on the average ED LOS, they recognized that ED patients and their families became disgruntled at some time limit past the average and that reducing the percentage of patients whose ED LOS exceeded this limit was much more meaningful than simply measuring the average; this concept is a central tenet of Lean Six Sigma. This approach especially appealed to senior leadership who customarily would hear complaints from those customers whose upper specification limit or tolerance had been exceeded (Caldwell et al. 2009). What better goal than to eliminate those outliers and horror stories of outrageous waits?

Based upon the external benchmarks, the three-year USL goal at Morton Plant was set at 250 minutes, or just over 4 hours. In the Lean Six Sigma strategy deployment approach, this means that the ED leadership was charged to redesign its critical subprocesses to assure that 99.9997 percent of ED patients were treated within 250 minutes. In other words, rather than focus on the average ED LOS, a Lean Six Sigma approach is to identify that point beyond which no patient should remain in the ED.

Accountability Structure

Rather than the more common Lean Six Sigma approach of completing one project, then deciding which project to do next, projects at Morton Plant and St. Vincent's were laid out in 100-day increments over a three-year period and were reevaluated at the end of each 100-day cycle. These projects, using the 100-Day Workout methodology, sought to execute quickly those changes in which an impact could be discerned within the 100-day implementation period. Figure 4.6 illustrates this strategic approach.

As discussed previously, the accountable structure should be separately managed from the use of Lean Six Sigma concepts and, in top quartile performers, is viewed as a nondelegable role of senior leaders and not left solely to Black Belts to manage. In the authors' research, top quartile performers designed their 100-Day Workout structures to assure presence of the following characteristics (Caldwell and Butler 2009):

■ An accountable vice president to organize and actively manage the accountability-based report-out process and not delegate this function to those lower

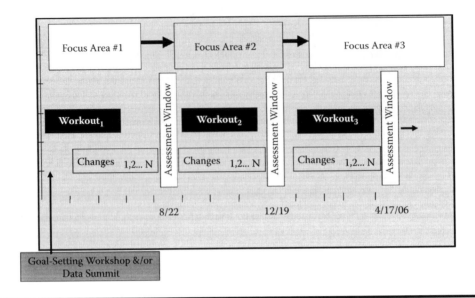

Figure 4.6 Rapid cycle test example. (Reproduced with permission from Caldwell and Butler, 2009.)

in the organization. This vice president keeps her/his eye on continuous improvement of the Big Q metric toward the three-year strategic goal and assures that each manager and Black Belt accomplishes those tasks necessary to achieve results.

■ Collaboration of two or more subprocess teams working simultaneously (but no more than five subprocess teams). These subprocess teams make up the Big Q ED continuum of care versus one ED-only subprocess team working by itself and in isolation, as illustrated by the St. Vincent's Big Q structure shown in Figure 4.2.

■ The expectation that each subprocess team present implementation of two successful process changes each month, preferably demonstrating that each change impacted the Big Q goal through the use of rapid cycle testing. The concept of rapid cycle testing will be reviewed in the next section on accelerating quality methods.

■ That the aforementioned successful process changes are presented in a public forum led by the accountable senior leader and attended by the CEO and other senior leaders.

The elements of a successful 100-Day Workout structure as found in the authors' published findings bear repetition. These elements are that, within a Big Q strategy deployment, the accountable vice president assures that at least two continuum-oriented subprocess teams work simultaneously in tandem, with each subprocess team expected to present results of two successful process changes in rapid cycle testing format each month in front of a public forum attended by the CEO, COO, or other senior leaders. Floyd Regional Medical Center CEO

Kurt Stuenkel, recognized as a top quartile performer in the authors' published work, announced during his speech at the 2008 annual meeting of the American College of Healthcare Executives that the combination of these elements far surpassed the use of Lean Six Sigma concepts in driving improvement work at his institution and that, moreover, the accountable structure was vital to assuring a sustainable improvement initiative (Stuenkel and Caldwell 2008).

At both Morton Plant and St. Vincent's, the first challenge of the senior management teams was to ensure that leadership within the ED, bed management, transportation, and nursing units were on board and recognized that Big Q results depended more upon their collaboration than upon their individualized, isolated efforts. The best-selling management book, *Good to Great,* by Collins (2001) lists this as a critical factor present in organizations that achieve quantum improvement. Care was taken to avoid polarizing the interests of the hospital and the physician groups.

Use of Accelerating Quality Concepts

The third and final leg of the three-legged top quartile stool is use of accelerating quality concepts like Lean Six Sigma. Although the authors' research found that those who viewed Lean Six Sigma as training alone risked organizational failure, the use of accelerating methods like Lean Six Sigma do just that—accelerate progress along the path to Big Q strategic results if utilized within an accountability structure as outlined in the previous section.

Most organizations have at some point in the recent past devoted significant time, energy, and, in many cases, significant consulting dollars, to improving the ED. Some have engaged Lean Six Sigma Black Belts only to achieve little q gains. Many of these organizations report frustration at achieving little q results (or none at all) or the inability to sustain short-term gains over the long haul. The causes of these frustrations can be multiple, but in each case, some of the frustration can be traced to the approaches utilized by the organization to prioritize improvement opportunities and to validate that changes truly resulted in ED LOS improvement.

Although the typical Lean Six Sigma toolkit possesses many tools and methods, the three most notable for accelerating improvement work are:

- Dramatically increasing the "speed to implementation" by improving the time effectiveness of the opportunity prioritization process
- Application of proven Lean change concepts versus the less effective trial and error of best practices or simple brainstorming
- By application of the concept of rapid cycle testing, validating that individual changes made by participating department managers and subprocess teams do indeed move the organization toward its three-year Big Q goal, both of which are reviewed in the following

Prioritizing Subprocess Improvement Opportunities

At the case study organizations, after determining the Big Q strategic USL and assigning the desired strategic goal to an accountable senior leader, the next task was to construct a high-level ED process flow, using the Lean Six Sigma supplier-input-process-output-customer (SIPOC) tool. The result of this activity was a validation that a limited number of critical subprocesses existed and, if synchronized and integrated, the probability of achieving the Big Q goal increased. That is, the use of the statistical prowess of Lean Six Sigma enabled these organizations to avoid the relatively unsuccessful improvement approach of best practices replication and trial and error, instead focusing on those vital few critical processes.

In Lean Six Sigma lingo, these vital few subprocesses are referred to colloquially as "critical Xs" and are usually the result of statistical multivariate regression analysis, although certified Black Belts have a number of tools in their toolkits to aid in the prioritization process. In both organizations, as well as most organizations researched by the authors, these critical subprocesses were in order of statistical impact:

- Time from the *last* diagnostic test order to result
- Time from patient entry to ED bed
- Time from ED bed to physician assessment
- Time from triage to first radiology order

The results of this prioritization activity are typically displayed in tabular format as illustrated in Table 4.2.

As will be observed by many readers, these subprocesses mirror those reported by many well-publicized ED process improvement efforts (Healthcare Advisory Board 1999). Yet the exercise of displaying the process flow and selecting the critical subprocesses to measure was important for buy-in by the individuals involved in the subprocess teams in both organizations. The use of statistical predictors has a most notable impact on physicians, who are accustomed to the use of statistical tools in their day-to-day work.

While considering the prioritization process discussed earlier, as commonly used in a Lean Six Sigma methodology suite, the reader will benefit from reflecting upon the broader notion of improvement opportunity prioritization. When thought of in this way, past efforts by organizations to improve Big Q processes can be affinitized into the following categories, presented in order of effectiveness (Caldwell et al. 2009):

- Shoot from the hip—Process change without any data to support the change concept is the most commonly observed approach. This "let's just do something" mentality seems to exist among physician teams as well as operations teams. It is as if physicians, once they leave the patient care areas, often totally abandon their scientific approach to clinical problem solving. No

Table 4.2 Data Summit Regression Analysis Table

	N	*Percent*	*Average*	*25th Percentile*	*Median*	*75th Percentile*	*95th Percentile*	*R²*
LOS (hr)	2472	100%	6.97	3.73	6.20	9.37	15.36	100%
LOS (min)	2472	100%	418	224	372	562	921	100%
Quick reg. to complete triage	2472	100%	27	9	17	34	75	5%
Triage to ED bed	2472	100%	127	16	70	193	436	47%
ED bed to MD assess	2472	100%	73	16	48	102	221	31%
ED reg to first lab order	1205	49%	112	45	78	135	340	23%
First lab order to verified	1228	50%	54	21	35	66	148	20%
Last lab verified to ED discharge	1354	55%	244	85	187	344	639	72%
ED reg to first radiology order	1369	55%	156	48	98	217	484	46%
First radiology order to last verified	1315	53%	68	17	37	86	231	23%
Last radiology verified to ED discharge	1401	57%	288	118	231	406	709	76%

Source: Reproduced with permission from Caldwell and Butler (2009). St. Vincent's ED data, 2006. N-2472

physician would treat a patient's pathophysiology without rigorous follow-up diagnostics to assure the therapeutic regimen was effective. Yet, inside an improvement meeting, teams sometimes throw all scientific logic out the window, searching for the first quick fix.

■ Trial and error of best practices—Utilizing improvement practices found in the literature, at meetings, or through benchmarking services like the Healthcare Advisory Board can provide a rich solution set for a team to brainstorm. However, application of these best practices without first understanding the major sources of variation within an organization's own processes can lead to wasted effort.

■ Simple regression analysis—In what the Lean Six Sigma project methodology refers to as critical-to-quality characteristics (CTQ), an effort is made to uncover those subprocesses that, if improved, will likely lead to improvement of overall Big Q performance. For example, at Morton Plant, it was discovered that if all tests could be ordered within 45 minutes, there was a significant probability that the total LOS would not exceed 250 minutes.

- Multivariate regression analysis—Similar to simple regression, multivariate regression analysis also examines the impact of more than one subprocess on overall Big Q performance.
- Small scale experiments—Using factorial analysis or simply run charting of only 25 data points (Langley et al. 1996, 110), teams can evaluate multiple process change concepts simultaneously by sampling just a few tests of change per day or shift to determine the optimum mix of change ideas. While small scale experiments are useful for improvement opportunity prioritization, it is also the underlying concept of rapid cycle testing discussed in the next section.
- Simulation—Simulation allows for the testing of potential improvements without actually going through the sometimes traumatic process of piloting. While expensive and conducted best by experienced statisticians and simulationists, simulation is particularly useful when throughput and staffing/ capacity optimization are key.

Hopefully, upon review of these improvement prioritization approaches, the reader will recognize the potential to avoid the often time-wasting impact of reliance upon shoot from the hip and trial and error of best practices approaches and seek to apply more time-effective and result-effective approaches.

Lean Change Concepts

Effective use of Lean within organizations can aid in their redesign logic versus the less effective trial and error of best practices or brainstorming alone. The Lean change concept library consists of the following (Caldwell and Butler 2009):

1. Develop contingency plans for failure modes
2. Consolidate functions/processes; eliminate steps
3. Initiate dependent subprocesses earlier in the process
4. Parallel process nondependent subprocesses
5. Decrease subprocess cycle times
6. Eliminate waste, errors, waits, and delays
7. Match staffing and capacity to demand
8. Shape demand

Although this abbreviated listing should provide readers with an intuitive sense of how Lean change concepts can provide more intellectual structure to its non-Lean approaches, full treatment of the 84 Lean change concepts is beyond the scope of this chapter. Readers who desire a more rich discussion of Lean application in health care are directed to the authors' textbook *Lean-Six Sigma for Healthcare* (Caldwell et al. 2009)

Rapid Cycle Testing Process

The technique of small-scale experiments, in addition to aiding in the improvement prioritization activities discussed earlier, is the underlying concept for rapid cycle testing. The idea of rapid cycle testing, while quite simple, is perhaps the most vital and most underutilized. In a rapid cycle testing framework, subprocess teams are asked to demonstrate the effectiveness of their two changes per month during the monthly public forum discussed in the accountable structure section.

The rapid cycle testing approach is straightforward enough. Subprocess teams report in graphic format baseline performance compared to the impact, if any, of their process change. Two examples of typical rapid cycle tests are illustrated in Figure 4.7 and Figure 4.8.

For more detailed treatment of the rapid cycle testing concept, the reader is directed to Caldwell et al. (2009).

Lean Six Sigma and Cost Recovery

Many readers, particularly senior leaders, will be interested in studying the relationship between Big Q ED LOS improvements and recovering costs associated with this throughput improvement. Process throughput, process cost, and cost recovery are interrelated, but not interdependent, as so many senior leaders have found. That is, by simply becoming more "lean," the organization will not necessarily recover associated costs without taking additional measures.

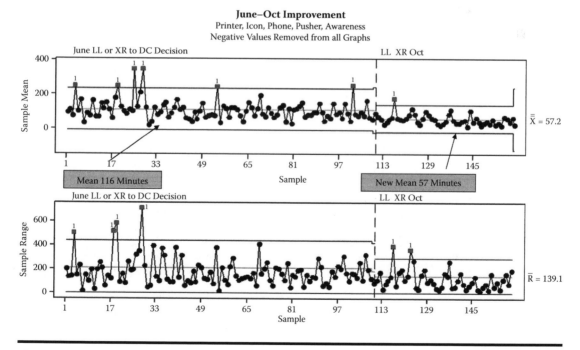

Figure 4.7   Rapid cycle test example. (Reproduced with permission from Caldwell and Butler, 2009.)

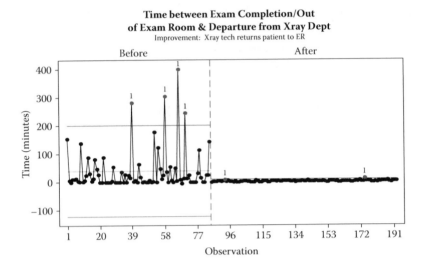

Figure 4.8   ED lab order to lab result improvement.

Mozena et al. (1999) notes that "costs are not causes," but rather symptoms of the interrelationships between and within processes. Not all process improvement opportunities will return cost recovery as the exhaust nor will all improvements yield cost recovery without additional activity on the part of leadership.

Generally, the following paradigm proves helpful in determining the additional effort required, if any, to extract cost from process throughput improvements:

■ Type 1—A process throughput improvement produces a direct cost recovery. For example, an ED LOS reduction can result in one or more of three types of savings. First, a significant reduction in diversion minutes is likely, producing additional incremental profit, with no new staffing. Second, patients leaving without treatment will decrease without any additional activity. And, third, a Type 2 savings occurs, worked hours per ED visit, explained next.

■ Type 2—A process throughput improvement that produces time saved, but no cost recovery without an additional action to impact worked hours per unit of service. As in the ED example earlier, two events will automatically occur under a Type 1 savings, requiring no action on the part of leadership, but one Type 2 savings results. This Type 2 savings is ED nurse worked hours per ED visit. If ED LOS averages 4 hours and ED worked hours per visit approach 3 hours per ED visit, then the department is investing 0.75 worked hours for every ED patient hour. As a throughput improvement concept, Lean Six Sigma thinking suggests that, as throughput improves, staff time is saved in the form of reduced staff worked hours per unit of service.

For example, if ED LOS decreases, which is a throughput improvement, staff time is saved in the form of reduced patient care hours required of ED staff. If ED LOS decreases 25 percent, to 3 hours, then 0.75 worked hours are freed up for every ED patient. However, these savings are not driven automatically to the bottom line without additional activity. In order to capitalize on this gained economy, the organization's leadership must reduce the hours during which selected ED rooms are staffed.

In other words, in a Type 2 savings, the demand curve on the ED will decrease significantly, but in order to recover any portion of these 0.75 worked hours per ED visit, the ED management must adjust the hours during which selected rooms are operational. It is important to note, however, that 100 percent of the conversion of time saved into reduced worked hours per unit of service is exceedingly rare. As a general rule of thumb, the organization can expect to recover between at least 50 percent of the time saved, but not more than 75 percent. (Caldwell et al. 2009).

Type 2 savings are the most common and, in fact, almost every department, with the proper training and Black Belt support, can derive significant cases of Type 2 savings. In the case of surgery, for example, if we are able to improve surgery throughput reducing hours per operating room case by 30 minutes, we only realize cost recovery if we are able to close selected operating rooms earlier in the day. Another example would be improving the rate of "noon discharge" percentage for inpatients so that over 80 percent of patients leave the inpatient setting by 2 p.m., just before shift change. In this case, the 3 p.m.–11 p.m. shift must be adjusted for the new evening shift patient demand. A third example would be reduced medical errors (including near misses). If nurses invest over 15 percent of their time inspecting and correcting medication errors and near misses, a 50-percent reduction in medication errors would produce at least 50 percent recovery of the time saved. However, capturing saved nurse time is a complicated process.

■ Type 3—A throughput savings improvement that produces optimized capacity. The underlying process throughput improvement for Type 3 savings is identical to Type 2 except that costs are recovered in the form of additional patients. In Type 2, worked hours per unit of service will decrease because staffed hours decrease. In Type 3 savings, worked hours per unit of service decrease because more patients are treated and released in the same staffed time. In our ED example earlier, we can convert our throughput improvement into a Type 3 savings if we can increase the number of patients treated, either through additional aggressive promotion or natural growth. In the case of surgery, for example, if we are able to improve surgery throughput reducing hours per operating room case by thirty minutes, we can capture Type 3 savings if we have surgeons willing to provide more cases because additional preferred surgery hours are available. Type 3 savings are by far the highest return on effort since we increase net revenue but incur almost no additional costs. However, Type 3 savings are less common, of course, unless the marketing department can drive additional volume or the organization's service area is experiencing a growth period.

When and How to Start the Journey

When to Start

The worst time to embrace Lean Six Sigma is when the organization is desperate or in trouble. Building a culture of high quality and process improvement is something the organization has an obligation to do because the staff and the patients deserve and expect it. Adopting Lean Six Sigma because senior leaders have tried every other approach without success is a little like starting to bail the boat when it is almost underwater. It is clearly better than doing nothing, but the best time to start would have been much sooner. Indeed, only those organizations enjoying top industry quality reputations and windfall profits could logically make an argument that it is not really a good time to embrace the philosophy and begin to explore the toolkit. Truth be known, most organizations enjoying that type of success have already adopted strategies like Lean Six Sigma.

How to Align the Team

First and most important, senior leaders must be fully committed to establishing high performance expectations within the organization and subsequently equipping administration and management with the proper tools to create those desired outcomes. Lean Six Sigma cannot just be something that lives inside a small department in the basement of the main corporate office building.

Many managers have experienced some type of organizational redevelopment, downsizing, employee value engineering, or reorganization that was rooted solely in an effort to reduce costs. Most of these initiatives were not grounded with any connection to the quality of the workflow. In many of their experiences, the value of a motivated and energized workforce in times of significant change was ignored. As a result of these types of poor experience, senior leaders need to be highly attuned to the sensitivities of the team members and ensure that all aspects of Lean Six Sigma are related back to the level of interaction between the patient and the staff. Part of that messaging, especially considering the failures of the past, is a reassurance that little q enhancements are ways to enhance a manager's ability to make budget instead of a means to further reduce the expense budget as improvements are identified. This focuses the new approach through a positive lens and allows the transition to be much less threatening for those who have lived through other experiences.

At the same time, team members are reassured the culture change is not a grab-and-run strategy to force unhealthy cost reductions; it must be well understood that senior leaders do expect a return on the investment. One very effective way to introduce this concept is with a frank discussion between C-level representatives and the management team. At Dr. P. Phillips, for example, the CEO described himself as the "tax man" and said from the very beginning that a portion of all savings would need to drop to the bottom line. The significance of the statement was that managers and administrators understood they would be able to retain their portion of the savings to be reinvested on the bench or at the bedside. In the ED, for example, efficiencies allowed registered nurses (RNs) to see more patients and spend a little more quality time with each one. The manager worked with the Black Belt to complete an in-quality staffing matrix, which made it possible to convert three open positions to two modified shift schedules, without giving up any resources currently deployed in the workforce.

Starting Slow (Being Patient)

Many organizations choose to begin the Lean Six Sigma journey with a special 100-day workout known as a waste walk. This very simple activity accomplishes many positive results in a relatively short period of time. The waste walk is especially effective at getting managers engaged and helping to identify those who have an aptitude for leadership in Lean Six Sigma. In larger organizations, a subset of the management team can be engaged in this important kick-off activity, while smaller organizations might bring the entire middle management team together and invest in training for everyone from the very beginning.

In the early phase of adoption, it is important to focus on standardizing processes so it will be evident how well the new culture is addressing the need for positive change. As the environment becomes more of a challenge at the same time that boards and customers have rising expectations, organizations need the kind of advantage a Lean Six Sigma culture creates.

Organize for Success

At Dr. P. Phillips Hospital, the Lean Six Sigma initiative reports directly to the COO, who is himself a Green Belt. The CEO, however, was the initial public advocate and continues to demonstrate a personal interest by communicating frequently with the program director and members of various project teams. It is critical for team members and managers to see Lean Six Sigma personnel as working at a high level of the organization. Top-level executives do not necessarily need to obtain formal Six Sigma credentials (Green Belt or Black Belt) to have credibility as executive sponsors. It is much more important for leaders to ensure that everyone in the organization knows they have a fundamental understanding of, personal belief in, and commitment to the principles and culture of Lean Six Sigma. Senior leaders maintain an optimum level of engagement and visibility as advocates of the methodology by openly engaging in prioritization of projects and attending report-outs where they can add credible feedback. A sound working knowledge can be achieved by spending time with the consultant or Black Belt to obtain an initial overview and supplementing with a modicum of literature review relevant to C-level executives. Periodic consultations with the Black Belt(s) will further ensure that the senior leader stays abreast of outputs and results, which will greatly enhance his or her credibility with affected parties, especially when addressing physician results and opportunities.

Next Steps

Organizations that have invested in Lean Six Sigma training and resources as well as organizations yet to embrace these accelerating quality concepts can dramatically increase their ED performance improvement efforts by taking these small but impactful next steps:

1. Leaders within organizations who are charged with quantum improvement of their ED can educate senior leaders regarding their nondelegable roles as described in this chapter, both for the purpose of aiding in ED improvement and as a means to improve the organization-wide quality improvement effectiveness.
2. Once engaged, senior leaders can analyze, either from internal resources or with outside assistance, their existing quality establishment, paying particular attention to their nondelegable roles, most notably assuring that Big Q versus little q strategic deployment and the effectiveness of the accountable implementation structure, which, again, cannot be managed by quality professionals and Black Belts alone as can the use of Lean Six Sigma concepts, but rather require the dedicated involvement of senior leaders.
3. In order to cease reliance on time wasting and frustrating "trial and error of best practices" improvement prioritization approach, organizations can acquire a Lean Six Sigma Big Q multivariate regression analysis as shown in this chapter. This Big Q continuum-based analysis as opposed to an ED-only focus not only demonstrates its importance to those influencers outside the ED, like hospitalists, bed management, and inpatient unit nurse managers, but also sets the stage for a broader-based accountability and ownership of ED improvement.
4. Through the utilization of the rapid cycle testing concept, organizations can provide better proof of effectiveness of each change's impact on Big Q progress, but also enables the organization to establish a more results-oriented culture.

Summary

The probability of achieving and sustaining Big Q strategic results in the ED can be dramatically increased—as well as assuring that the time and resources devoted to the improvement effort—through the judicious application of the three elements of Big Quality versus little quality, senior leader-driving accountability structure, and effective application of accelerating quality concepts like Lean Six Sigma. To realize these benefits, however, senior leaders must recognize their nondelegable roles and assure effectiveness of their involvement.

References

Butler, Greg, and Chip Caldwell. 2008. *What Top-Performing Healthcare Organizations Know: 7 Proven Steps for Accelerating and Achieving Change.* Chicago: Health Administration Press.

Caldwell, Chip, and Greg Butler. September 17–18, 2009. "Improving Throughput and Costs Using Lean Six Sigma." Conference presented for American College of Healthcare Executives, Honolulu, HI.

Caldwell, Chip, Greg Butler, and Nancy Poston. 2009. *Lean Six Sigma for Healthcare: A Senior Leader Guide to Improving Cost and Throughput,* 2nd ed. Milwaukee, WI: ASQ Quality Press.

Collins, Jim. 2001. *Good to Great.* New York: HarperCollins.

Ford, Kathie. 2007. "Embracing Six Sigma-Third Wave Completed." In *100-Day Quality Workout, Wave III,* edited by Kathie Ford, 2. Jacksonville, FL: St. Vincent's Healthcare.

Healthcare Advisory Board. 1999. *The Clockwork ED.* Washington: Advisory Board Company.

Langley, Gerald, Kevin Nolan, Thomas Nolan, Clifford Norman, and Lloyd Provost. 1996. *The Improvement Guide.* San Francisco: Jossey-Bass.

Morton Plant Hospital. 2008. http://www.mortonplant.com/body.cfm?id=421 (accessed July 22, 2008).

Mozena, James, Charles Emerick, and Steven Black. 1999. *Stop Managing Costs.* Milwaukee, WI: ASQ Quality Press, 17.

Pieper, Shannon. 2004. "Good to Great in Healthcare." *Healthcare Executive* 19(3): 21–26.

St. Vincent's Medical Center. 2008. About Us. http://www.jaxhealth.com/AboutUs/default.asp?ENOrgID=17A49CA7DF5E416CA5C19C32F97C2210 (accessed July 22, 2008).

Stuenkel, Kurt, and Chip Caldwell. March 10–11, 2008. "The Senior Leaders Role in Throughput and Cost Recovery." Presented at the American College of Healthcare Executives annual meeting, Chicago.

Chapter 5

Queuing Models for Hospital Emergency Departments

Yasar A. Ozcan

Introduction

The American emergency medical system (EMS) has struggled since its inception to remain true to its original mission to handle emergent cases. Initially a site of acute care, the emergency department (ED) has quickly become a site where nonurgent, urgent, and acute cases meet with few options for patients and providers alike to seek alternative and perhaps even more appropriate care. As a result, patients of all acuity levels present to the ED (McCaig and Nawar, 2006). A major policy intervention in the history of emergency medicine was the passage of the Emergency Medical Treatment and Active Labor Act (EMTALA) in 1986. This prevented hospitals from refusing to treat patients or transferring them to charity or county hospitals because they are unable to pay or covered under Medicare or Medicaid. Enforced by the federal government, EMTALA poses two requirements on hospitals: (1) a hospital must provide an appropriate medical screening exam to anyone who comes to the ED and requests care, and (2) if the ED determines the person has an emergency medical condition, appropriate stabilization treatment and hospitalizations as necessary must be provided. The passage of EMTALA quickly poised the ED to become an integral component of the U.S. health care safety net (Hadley and Cunningham, 2004; Siegel, 2004).

The ED became no longer a place only for episodic care, where serious illness and injury were acutely addressed. Today, emergency medicine operates at the intersection of medical care, public health, and public safety (Institute of Medicine [IOM], 2006). The 2006 IOM report "Hospital-Based Emergency Care: At the Breaking Point" summarizes the new role of the ED perhaps most appropriately:

1. ED is a refuge to the 45 million uninsured in the USA.
2. ED becomes a valuable practice asset to the community physicians who channel complicated cases (risk aversion) to abundant technology choices available in ED.
3. ED is a convenient, one-stop shopping for the patient—always available, faster than going to physician office with appointment.
4. ED became an escape valve to the hospital for its strained inpatient capacity through holding units.

EDs receive an almost steady stream of patients. If an individual arriving by ambulance cannot be transferred quickly to an ED stretcher, efficiently triaged, and then rapidly evaluated, stabilized, and admitted or discharged, ED crowding will quickly develop, and patient care will be compromised. To handle specific urgent care, many EDs developed triage protocols for stroke patients, neurotrauma, hyperbaric, burn, eye, perinatal, and hand centers. In parallel to this, EDs developed fast track care, which is a dedicated area in or next to the ED that is specifically designed and designated for patients with minor illnesses or injuries. It is typically staffed by midlevel providers, such as physician assistants and nurse practitioners, working under the supervision of an emergency physician. Fast tracks can operate during regular business hours or during the ED's busiest times (e.g., evenings and weekends). Currently, fast tracks are in place at roughly 30 percent of all EDs, with approximately 30 percent of presenting patients being routed to these areas for care (Joint Commission, 2004; Wilson and Nguyen, 2004).

Nevertheless, a patient arriving at an ED must first be evaluated for the seriousness of his/her condition to be appropriately triaged. We can conceptualize arriving patients forming a queue based on this triage. Figure 5.1 depicts this

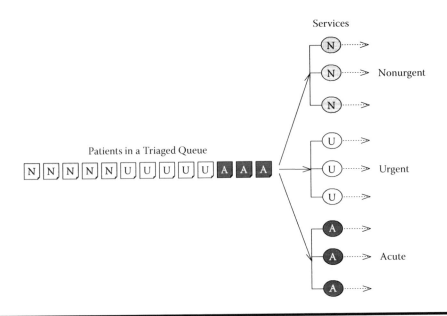

Figure 5.1   Emergency department triage.

conceptualization where patients triaged into three groups of seriousness (priorities), namely, acute, urgent, and nonurgent. This conceptualization assumes that patients with the highest priority (urgent) will be served first. However, within each priority category, there would be waiting line where patients may be handled based on first-come, first-served basis. Queuing theory provides an approach to evaluate performance of the system handling the patients who form a waiting line.

Queuing Theory

Queuing theory is a mathematical approach to the analysis of waiting lines. Waiting lines in health care organizations can be found wherever either patients or customers arrive randomly for services, such as ED arrivals (Ozcan, 2005).

The following example illustrates why patients must wait in lines. A hospital ED may have the capacity to handle an average of 40 patients an hour, and yet may have waiting lines even though the average number of patients is only 25 an hour. The key word is average. In reality, patients arrive at random intervals rather than at evenly spaced intervals, and some patients require more intensive treatment (longer service time) than others. In other words, both arrivals and length of service times exhibit great variability. As a result, the ED becomes temporarily overloaded at times, and patients have to wait. One way to resolve this problem is to increase capacity. Note that as service capacity increases, so does its cost. As capacity increases, however, the number of patients waiting and the time they wait tend to decrease, as do the performance measures of the ED. The goal of the queuing analysis is to identify the level of service capacity that will minimize costs and improve service performance.

An ED manager can choose from among a few queuing models. Choosing the appropriate one is the key to solving the problem successfully. Model choice depends on the characteristics of the ED. The main queuing model characteristics are: (1) the population source, (2) queue discipline, (3) number of servers, and (4) arrival and service rates.

Population source is the first characteristic to look at when analyzing a queuing problem. Consider whether the potential number of patients is limited, that is, whether the population source is infinite or finite. In an infinite source situation, patient arrivals are unrestricted and can greatly exceed system capacity at any time. An infinite source exists when service (access) is unrestricted, such as with an ED.

Queue discipline refers to the order in which customers are processed. The general assumption that service is provided on a first-come, first-served basis is probably the most commonly encountered rule. However, in the emergency department, a first-come basis is not appropriate. Patients do not all represent the same risk; those with the highest risk (acute) are processed first under a triage system, even though other patients may have arrived earlier. Figure 5.1 depicts a triage system for an ED where patients are grouped into three categories of

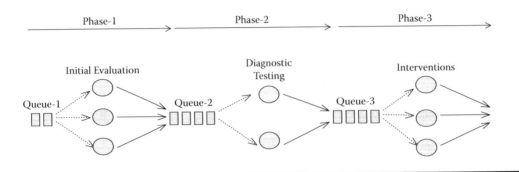

Figure 5.2 Multiline, multiphase queues in an emergency department.

risk: acute, urgent, and nonurgent. In this case, the ED may be conceptualized as offering three different service lines.

The next question is how many servers are needed to run the ED appropriately. The number of servers determines the capacity of queuing systems. It is generally assumed that each server can handle one patient at a time. An ED can be conceptualized as multiple line and may consist of phases. Although the phases will vary from patient to patient, because each one receives care from several staff members in succession, the configuration in this case is a multiple-line queuing system. Figure 5.2 illustrates the multiple-line, multiphase queuing example.

Determination of capacity depends on patient arrivals (arrival rate) and service speed (service rate).

ED queues are generally owed to randomness, highly variable arrival and service patterns that cause systems to be temporarily overloaded. Hospital EDs are very typical examples of erratic arrival patterns causing such variability. The arrival patterns might be different on mornings and afternoons, and even more so after physician offices close in the evenings. In general, queues are more prevalent in evening hours and on weekends. Besides that, in any block of time there are no discernible patterns, so the random nature of the arrivals—their numbers and the times between the arrivals—has to be measured. The variability can often be described by theoretical distributions. The most commonly used models assume that the patient arrival rate can be described by a Poisson distribution. On the other hand, service to the arriving patients is another element that exhibits variability. Because of the varying nature of illnesses and patient conditions, the time required for clinical attention (service times) varies from patient to patient. The service rate and service times are also interchangeably used, so that the Poisson distribution can characterize the service rate. If arrival rates are more than service rates, then a multichannel queue system is appropriate

Before describing such models, one needs to identify the performance measures that would guide managers for better management (of capacity) for the ED.

λ: arrival rate
μ: service rate

L_q: average number of customers waiting for service

L: average number of customers in the system (waiting or being served)

W_q: average time customers wait in line

W: average time customers spend in the system

ρ: system utilization

P_0: probability of zero patients in system

Assuming patients are triaged appropriately, queuing problems in an ED can be solved using various methodologies. One methodology is to solve each triaged group as a separate problem using a multiserver queuing method (Ozcan, 2005). Another method is a multiple-priority model. However, the model with multiple priorities makes strong assumptions on how the patients will be called from the queue. That is, patients are assigned to priority classes (e.g., nonurgent, urgent, and acute), then patients in the highest class (acute) are treated first. When there is no one left within the acute queue, then urgent patients followed by nonurgent patients would be treated. However, this model assumes that if another urgent or emergent patient arrives, it takes priority over the lesser priority class patients. The patients within the same priority class would be treated on a first-come, first-served basis. In addition, average treatment times for each class (service rate) are often assumed to be the same for each priority class.

Modifying this assumption to assign differing service rates to each priority class further complicates the formulations (Stevenson, 2006). Nevertheless, using the multiple-priority formulation for emergency services does not reflect exactly what takes place in contemporary EDs. Fast tracks and other processes that separate the ED patient population is more amenable to solving queuing problems independently for each type of category. Of course this has its own assumptions that nonurgent, urgent, and acute are considered as independent service lines. Figure 5.2 further illustrates the conceptualization of a multiline, multiphase system as a continuation of Figure 5.1, and this is typical for the ED environment, especially for nonurgent and urgent cases. After triage, patients reach a medical professional for initial medical evaluation, then they enter a queue for diagnostic tests (second queue), and finally they move into an intervention stage for treatment (third queue).

The Queuing Model

Given the previous assumptions, solving ED queuing problems with separate (partitioned) queuing models would simplify the solutions for ED managers. In the remainder of this chapter we will demonstrate how such solutions can be easily attained using an example and provide the solutions using an Excel template.

Queuing analysis formulations for multiserver models require intensive formulations for queue length (L_q) and idle system (P_0):

$$L_q = \frac{\lambda\mu\left(\frac{\lambda}{\mu}\right)^s}{(s-1)!(s\mu-\lambda)^2}P_0$$

$$P_0 = \frac{1}{\left[\sum_{n=0}^{s-1}\frac{\left(\frac{\lambda}{\mu}\right)^n}{n!} + \frac{\left(\frac{\lambda}{\mu}\right)^s}{s!\left(1-\frac{\lambda}{s\mu}\right)}\right]}$$

In multiserver models, two additional performance measures can be calculated as:

$$W_a = \frac{1}{s\mu-\lambda}$$

$$P_w = \frac{W_q}{W_a}$$

where
  W_a = the average time for an arrival not immediately served, and
  P_w = probability that an arrival will have to wait for service.

Measures of Queuing System Performance

The ED manager must consider four typical measures when evaluating existing or proposed service systems. Those measures are:

1. Average number of patients waiting (in queue or in the system)
2. Average time the patients wait (in queue or in the system)
3. Capacity utilization
4. Probability that an arriving patient will have to wait for service

The system utilization measure reflects the extent to which the servers are busy rather than idle. On the surface, it might seem that ED managers would seek 100 percent system utilization. However, increases in system utilization are achieved only at the expense of increases in both the length of the waiting line and the average waiting time for all patients, with values becoming exceedingly large as utilization approaches 100 percent. Under normal circumstances,

100 percent utilization may not be realistic; an ED manager should try to achieve a system that provides an acceptable wait time in queue and utilization between 75 percent and 90 percent. In queue modeling, the ED manager also must ensure that average arrival and service rates are stable, indicating that the system is in a steady state, a fundamental assumption.

An Example of Emergency Department Performance Evaluation

Hand-solving multiline queuing problems are beyond both the intent of this text and the time available to health care managers. However, using an Excel queuing template that incorporates these formulas, one can employ such higher order models for their capacity formulations and for measuring existing and redesigned systems' performance. To illustrate the concepts defined earlier and to provide a working tool for ED managers to evaluate performance of the ED, an example with an ED scenario is presented next.

ED Scenario

Emergency department services in ABC Hospital peak on weekends. Historically, the ED has provided space for five stations (examining rooms) for nonemergency cases, three stations for urgent case, and two stations for acute cases during weekends. Nonemergency patients are examined on a first-come, first-served basis, and urgent and acute cases are treated on a most serious, first-served basis, after a triage nurse has screened all cases. The ED currently experiences congestion, especially for urgent and acute cases, and the ED manager wants to know how additional resources in the ED might reduce congestion and waiting times.

The past year's operating data were gathered from the information systems; they included records of arrival and service times. Preliminary examination of the data revealed little seasonal variation in ED use for that year, and ED personnel stated that their protocols and procedures had remained relatively constant.

The arrival pattern of patients, tabulated for weekends during last year (total of 2,500 hours), showed that 22,500 nonemergency, 7,500 urgent, and 3,750 acute patients came to the ED during that time. The arrival pattern approximates a Poisson distribution. After a lengthy time-motion study, the average service time was found to be 30 minutes per nonemergency, 60 minutes for urgent, and 120 minutes for acute patients.

Solution to the ED Congestion Problem

Since there are three different service lines based on triage, arrival and service rates need to be determined separately for each service line. Arrival rate is determined as the average arrivals for a given time period; there are 22,500 nonurgent arrivals during 2,500 weekend hours. Thus, we could establish that the average arrival rate is 9 (22,500 ÷ 2,500 = 9) nonurgent patients per hour. Arrival rate for urgent patients during this period is similarly determined to be 3 (7,500 ÷ 2,500 = 3); and finally, arrival rate for the acute patients assessed as 1.5 (3,750 ÷ 2,500 = 1.5).

Service rate can be calculated based on how many patients can be served in a time period. Since we used 1 hour (60 minutes) as the nomenclature to calculate the arrival rates, service rates should be based on a similar metric. Hence the average service rate for nonurgent patients is 2 (60 ÷ 30 = 2), for urgent patients it is 1 (60 ÷ 60 = 1), and for acute patients it is 0.5 (60 ÷ 120 = 0.5). The next question for the ED manager is what are the system performance measures for this situation.

The Excel template (available from author: ozcan@vcu.edu) can be used to generate alternative solutions. Based on calculated rates of arrival (λ) and service (μ) for each service line—nonurgent, urgent, and acute—the ED manager can explore various capacity alternatives by examining various performance measures discussed earlier and available from the template. To evaluate alternative solutions for each service line, Excel templates require only that arrival (λ) and service (μ) rates and the current or future capacity (*s*) information be entered in the highlighted areas of the spreadsheet. Excel template solutions are provided in Figures 5.3 through 5.5 for this example. Results shown on the left part of the each figure provide the solution for the current capacity for each of the service lines, and the right portion of each figure shows an acceptable solution to the existing situation.

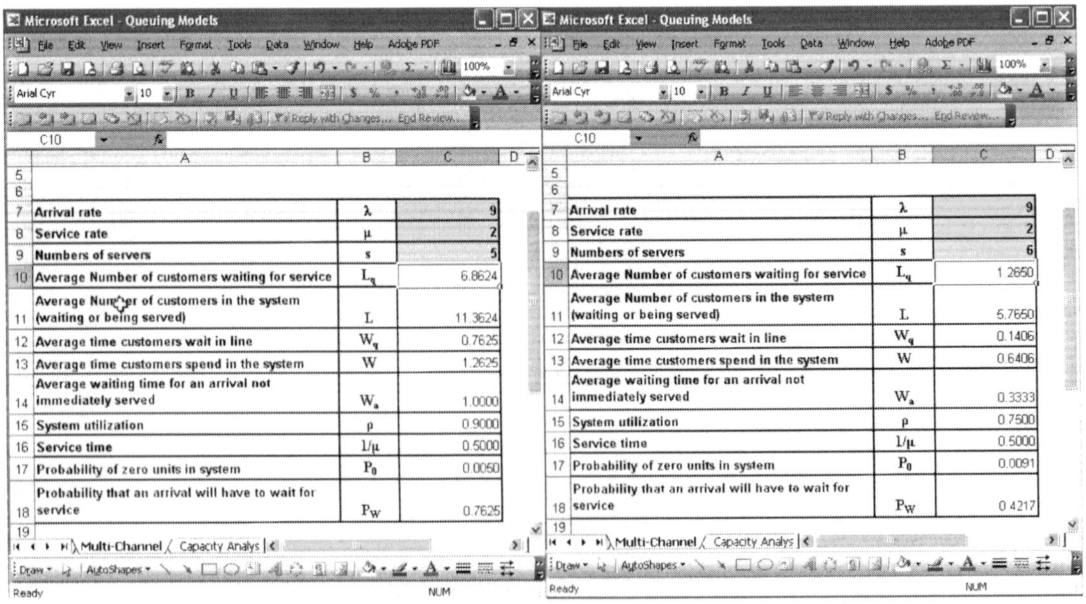

Figure 5.3   Performance measures for nonurgent service line; five and six stations.

Nonurgent Service Line

As shown in Figure 5.3, the current service capacity is five servers and the system utilization (ρ) is at 90 percent. On average there are about 6.86 (L_q) nonurgent patients waiting to be served and their wait time (W_q) is about 0.7625 hours, or approximately 45 minutes (0.7625 × 60 = 45.75). About 11.36 (L) patients are in the system, and from entry to exit nonurgent patients spend about 1.2625 hours (or 75 minutes) in the system. We can also deduce that there are 4.5 (11.36 – 6.86 = 4.5) nonurgent patients being served during the weekend hours. It is noteworthy to observe that a low probability of zero units in the system (P_0) would indicate a high utilization or that the system is near full capacity. Hence, the ED manager can explore the capacity increase for the ED by one station, for a total of six stations, and observe the impact on performance. The probability that a newly arriving patient (P_w) has to wait is 0.76, indicating that the length of a queue (L_q) and wait time (W_q) will be longer.

The solution presented on the right-hand portion of Figure 5.3 provides insight to this situation, where utilization drops to 75 percent. But wait time is now only about 8 minutes. In such a situation, the ED manager may want to stay with the status quo for the nonurgent patient service line, unless there is likely to be an increase in arrival rate in the future.

Urgent Service Line

The situation for the urgent service line is more problematic as shown in the left part of Figure 5.4, where utilization is at 100 percent; thus the system is unstable

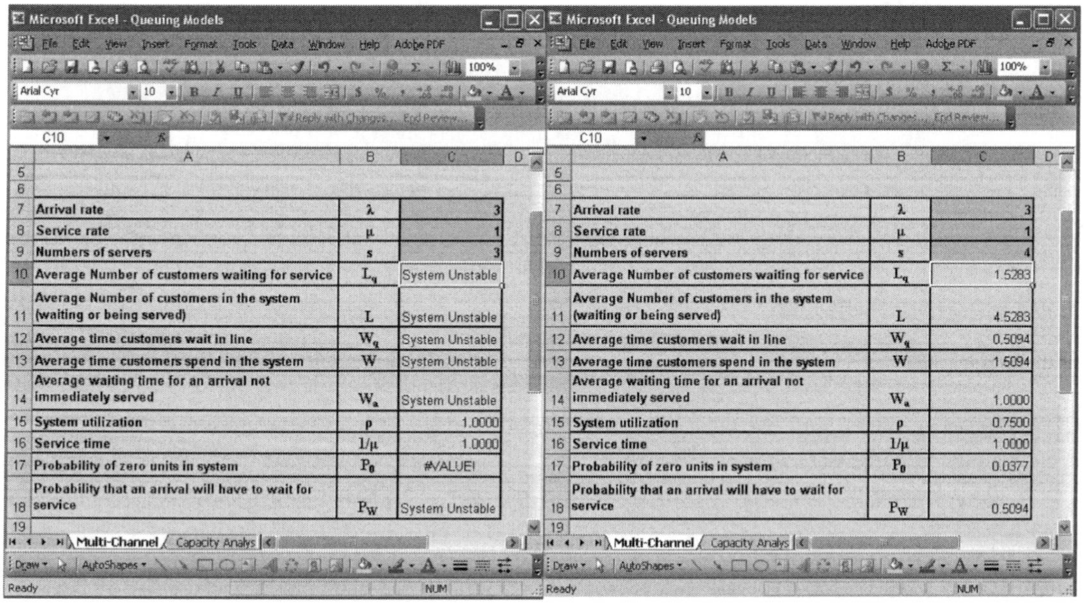

Figure 5.4   Performance measures for urgent service line; three and four stations.

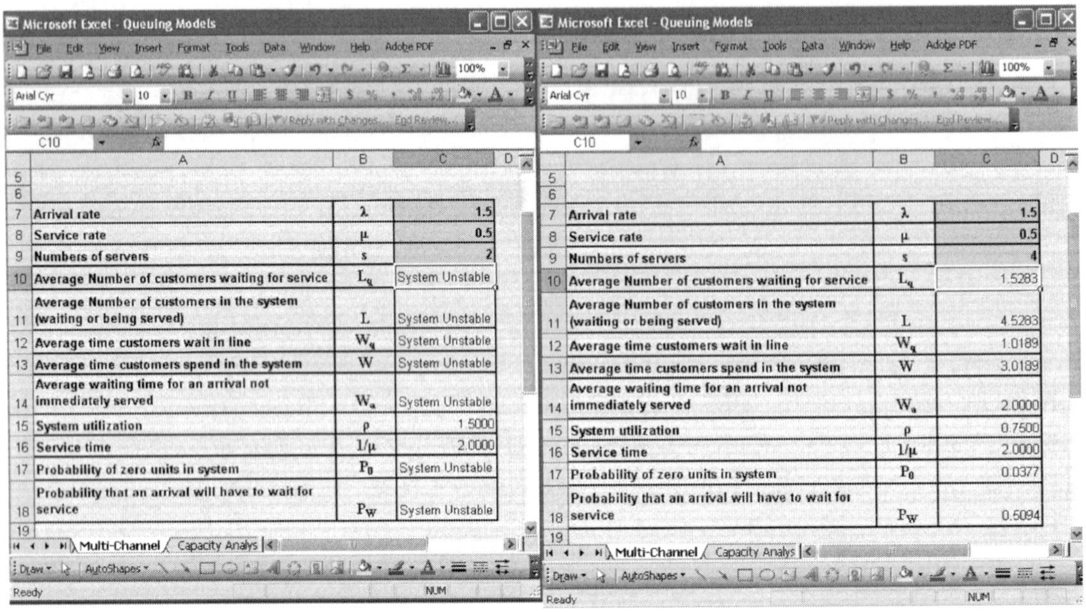

Figure 5.5   Performance measures for acute service; two and four stations.

to handle the urgent patients using only three stations. However, an additional station on this service line (four servers), as shown on the right portion of Figure 5.4, provides reasonable performance measures at a 75-percent utilization rate. Urgent patients would only have to wait about 30 minutes ($W_q = 0.5094$).

Acute Service Line

The acute case service line currently has only two stations (servers) and the situation is more dramatic than with the other ED service lines. The utilization is 150 percent and the system is unstable (see the left portion of Figure 5.5). Thus, a definite capacity increase is needed. Adding an extra station does not solve the problem for this situation, thus two extra stations (servers) need to be added (see the right portion of Figure 5.5). This would bring the utilization down to 75 percent and the wait time to approximately one hour. In lieu of utilization, the ED manager might want to further increase the resources (servers) to reduce wait times for acute patients.

Summary

The realities of emergency departments can be abstracted and analyzed using queuing models. The key to this abstraction is to identify the bottleneck in operations and evaluate that portion of the operation. An emergency department may be responding to the needs of patients adequately during weekdays, but difficulties may be arising over the weekends and in certain hours of the evening.

Queue discipline is a factor especially important in emergency departments. ED managers must look at the condition and risk of the arriving patient, and process patient service according to acute, urgent, and least urgent care through the triage process. As shown earlier, the corresponding problem can be evaluated as separate (partitioned) problems in queuing situations—with varying arrival and service rates. That is, even in the same ED system, queue problems can be identified for different categories of patients.

References

Emergency Medical Treatment and Active Labor Act (EMTALA). (1986). U.S. Code 42 § 1395dd.

Hadley, J., and Cunningham, P. (2004). Availability of safety net providers and access to care of uninsured persons. *Health Services Research* 39(5): 1527–1546.

Institute of Medicine (IOM). (2006). *Hospital-Based Emergency Care: At the Breaking Point*. Washington DC: Institute of Medicine.

Joint Commission. (2004). Critical Access Hospitals—Fast Track. http://www.jointcommission.org/AccreditationPrograms/CriticalAccessHospitals/.

McCaig, L.F., and Nawar, E.W. (2006). *National Hospital Ambulatory Medical Care Survey: 2004 Emergency Department Summary*. Advance Data (No. 372). Hyattsville, MD: National Center for Health Statistics.

Ozcan, Y.A. (2005). *Quantitative Methods in Health Care Management: Techniques and Applications*. San Francisco: Jossey-Bass/Wiley.

Siegel, D.M. (2004). Healthcare reform: responding to the rhetoric. *Ostomy Wound Management* 50(11): 6–10.

Stevenson, W.J. (2006). *Operations Management* (8th ed.). New York: McGraw-Hill/Irwin.

Wilson, M., and Nguyen, K. September 2004. *Bursting at the Seams: Improving Patient Flow to Help America's Hospitals*. Washington, DC: Urgent Matters, The George Washington University Medical Center.

Chapter 6

The Nursing Perspective and Role in Planning a Simulation Modeling Project:

Historical, Experiential, and Future Applications of Complex Adaptive Systems Thinking

Susan O'Hara

Introduction

Health care is in crisis. Health care costs continue to rise, while medical errors have become the eighth leading cause of death in the United States (Institute of Medicine [IOM 2000]). A worsening nursing shortage has not improved despite mandated nurse-to-patient ratios (Anderson, 2007). Demographic trends threaten to worsen this crisis; as the U.S. population ages, patient acuity will increase, while the supply of working-age nurses will shrink (U.S. Census Bureau, 2000). A focus on nursing is an essential part of any potential solution to this looming problem. As a large body of literature clearly demonstrates, nurses are inextricably linked to patient outcomes. In short, more nurse hours per patient day are associated with reduced in-hospital mortality (Aiken et al., 1994, 1998, 2002a, 2002b).

Unfortunately, nurses are challenged to prioritize precious patient-care time against management commitments to new processes directed at improving efficiency and care quality. When not collecting data, testing new theories, or learning and implementing new technologies, the nurse is required to maximize time with patients. How is this possible? Currently, it is not. Nurses are choosing to leave the hospital, if not the profession, while patients see less of the nurses who remain at the bedside. According to a recent national time and motion study conducted by Hendrich et al. (2008), medical-surgical nurses spend only 30 percent of their time in the patient room, while activities such as documentation, medication administration, and care coordination outweigh direct patient time.[1] The authors suggest that inefficiencies in the nurse work environment, including technologies, work processes, and the physical space, detract from direct patient-care time.

Nurses enter the profession to care for patients. One experienced nurse, when interviewed as part of a simulation modeling initiative, summed up her frustration in one sentence. "I just want to do what I do best—take care of my patient," she said. To facilitate nurses' desire to nurse, they must clearly communicate, in a quantifiable manner, the issues and problems they face. To better understand the big picture, and to communicate with their administrations, nurses must incorporate systems thinking and the necessary data to support their complaints and instincts.

The multilayered inefficiencies in the nurse work environment revealed by the time and motion study may owe their genesis, at least in part, to a lack of systems thinking. The interconnected and complex nature of health care confounds solutions that do not adequately address these features of the system. Indeed, a nascent literature has developed in recent years describing health care as a complex adaptive system (CAS; Begun et al., 2003; Holden, 2005). In this concept, nurses are agents within the hospital system that act in interdependent but not always predictable ways.

The systems thinking required to reengineer patient-care processes and the physical space in which they are delivered requires an objective, "cross-cultural" toolset that grasps the complex nature of the nursing unit within measurable constraints, limitations, barriers, metrics, and outcomes. Simulation modeling represents such a tool. This chapter describes the nurse work environment as a complex adaptive system, and illustrates the role for simulation modeling in improving the efficiency and effectiveness of nursing care. This chapter also offers a nursing perspective for working on a simulation modeling project (using an ED case study) and ends with some thoughts about the future of simulation modeling to improve patient care and the nurse work environment.

The Role and Relevance of Nursing

Florence Nightingale said, "Nursing is the act of utilizing the environment of the patient to assist him in his recovery." This is a powerful statement that identifies *clinical* and *operational process* (engineering) thinking ("nursing is the act of …

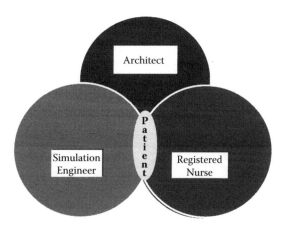

Figure 6.1   Patient Centered Modeling and Simulation Team.

to assist him in his recovery") and the role of architecture on patient care ("utilizing the environment").

The environment of care (the physical space), and the clinical and engineering approach to processes cannot be evaluated in isolation from one another. Professionals must fully understand not only the whole system through their own domain but must integrate their equal partners' domains to improve the system.

The nurse, as caregiver, has the greatest opportunity and challenge to provide simulation engineers and architects the comprehensive view on how to improve patient-care processes within the existing or proposed physical space (see Figure 6.1). The nurse as subject matter expert has a responsibility to the patient to ensure that improvement (and optimal care) is within a system and not simply through a component of that system.

Thus the first step of understanding a complex system is to understand the care processes, the caregivers, and the care environment. But is it that simple?

Complex adaptive systems thinking in nursing began with the work that Florence Nightingale did when she studied the role of processes in an environment. Triage, hand washing, and isolation process improvements within a crises environment (and facility) could and did decrease patient mortality.

As simple as this hypothesis sounds, it was a landmark concept. With help from the architects and engineers, she redesigned the floor plan of the wartime hospitals and the processes carried out within that redesign. She studied the behaviors of nurses and removed nurses from her team who made poor decisions or did not uphold the attributes of the nurses. (I visited the Florence Nightingale Museum in London, where I had the opportunity to read her staffing logs and annotations. She details the rationale for dismissing nurses such as drinking or staying out late. The staffing log also includes notes from Nightingale on nurses who may not have met the entrance training requirements, but provided excellent nursing care and were therefore not dismissed.)

Although she did not label her approach as simulation modeling, agent-based simulation, or CAS thinking, it is clear Nightingale used this approach. In many respects her "simulation" of the as-is conditions were founded in retrospective and real-time data collection, outcome documentation and measurement, and applied testing of what-if scenario thinking to her caregivers, care processes, and care environment. These simulations of the complex system in which she worked demonstrated both as-is conditions and what-if scenario testing and implementation, all within a CAS approach.

Since that time, nursing scholars have proven that CAS thinking can and does occur in the nursing environment. Although this chapter is not able to offer a detailed review of CAS, we offer a brief overview. It is recommended that the reader explore this topic in detail.

Baseline definitions and initial use of CAS follow. Next, a review of the nursing profession's application of CAS and complexity theory for the purpose of improving patient care is offered.

Nursing and Complex Adaptive Systems Thinking: Introduction

Complex adaptive systems are within the umbrella of complexity science. In the book, *Managing Business Complexity*, authors Michael North and Charles Macal explain the basic concepts: "Complexity science is a field that focuses on the universal principles common to all systems. Physical systems, emphasizing universal principles, as well as biological systems, emphasizing adaptation and emergence, are in the focus. Issues such as information, entropy, emergence, and how these arise from 'bottom up' principles are questions central to complexity science" (2007, 46). They go on to describe order and disorder in the universe (for our purposes the universe is the health care system). "One of the fundamental physical laws of nature is that disorder, that is, entropy, in the universe is constantly increasing. If disorder is increasing, how is it that systems can self-organize, effectively increasing order (i.e. decreasing disorder) in the universe? Such questions among others are the province of complexity science."

A quick overview of complex adaptive systems from Wikipedia:

> A CAS is a complex, self-similar collection of interacting adaptive agents. The study of CAS focuses on complex, emergent and macroscopic properties of the system. Various definitions have been offered by different researchers:
>
> ■ John H. Holland
>
> A Complex Adaptive System (CAS) is a dynamic network of many agents (which may represent cells, species, individuals, firms, nations) acting in parallel, constantly acting and reacting to what the other agents are doing. The control of a CAS tends to be highly dispersed and decentralized. If there is to be any coherent behavior

in the system, it has to arise from competition and cooperation among the agents themselves. The overall behavior of the system is the result of a huge number of decisions made every moment by many individual agents.

According to Holland himself, "The complex systems that I was interested in were those whose parts not only interacted to create novel properties, but also coevolved and adapted new rules to weather the fluctuations in their environment. I called them 'complex adaptive systems' or CAS." (CAS Group Blog/complex Adaptive Systems Group at http://blog.cas-group.net/?p=174).

"Emergence is a regular phenomenon in *complex adaptive systems* (*CAS*). A *CAS* consists of a large number of interacting individuals, called *agents*, which adapt or learn as they interact. Examples, with the corresponding agents in parentheses, are: markets (traders), ecosystems (organisms), the immune system (antibodies), biological cells (proteins), and so on. Some of our most complex current problems center on *CAS*:

- strengthening the immune system (antibodies)
- preserving ecosystems (organisms)
- understanding the evolution and acquisition of language (humans)
- controlling spam, viruses, and other intrusions on the Internet (sites)
- encouraging innovation in dynamic economies (firms)
- predicting the effects of trade laws on global trade (governments)" (From July 2007 discussion with Holland at http://www.pbs.org/wgbh/nova/sciencenow/3410/03-ask.html)

To continue the Wikipedia entry:

■ Kevin Dooley

A CAS behaves/evolves according to three key principles: order is emergent as opposed to predetermined (c.f. Neural Networks), the system's history is irreversible, and the system's future is often unpredictable. The basic building blocks of the CAS are agents. Agents scan their environment and develop schema representing interpretive and action rules. These schema are subject to change and evolution.

■ Other definitions

Macroscopic collections of simple (and typically nonlinearly) interacting units that are endowed with the ability to evolve and adapt to a changing environment.

The elements that make up a CAS are called agents. Not all simulation models require inclusion of agents. But all modeling projects are most successful if complex thinking is used. Providing the simulation engineers information using the complex thinking allows the simulation engineers to better scope the modeling approach. There are times that the modeling approach must be altered based on the information available. Giving the engineers a whole system overview of the process to be modeled allows them to better direct their input efforts to achieve the outcomes being studied. Selection of the individual components of a complex system as well as their contextual relationships to adjacent work environments or their integration into complimentary process can be discussed at the beginning of a model project.

Later we review the nursing perspective of building a process model (an ED case study) and the future of systems thinking in an agent-based health care model.

Nursing and Complex Adaptive Systems Thinking

Complex adaptive systems thinking has been used in various branches of health care and with simulation modeling tool sets. This chapter cannot attempt to cover all the models and papers, but the reader is referred to the Lancaster University Management School Working Paper 2007/003 by Adrian Fletcher and Dave Worthington titled "What Is a Generic Hospital Model?"

Nursing theorists have also adopted and adapted complex systems thinking to multiple nursing domains and clinically focused areas of practice. Applying theories to simulation modeling requires a brief overview of the theories. I have selected this succinct summary from "Extracts from Northern Arizona University; NUR 301: Perspectives in Professional Nursing" described by Evelyn Wilkerson (http://jan.ucc.nau.edu/~erw/nur301/index.html). This excerpt offers the most concise global view necessary to meet the requirements of this chapter.

> Theory can be defined as "an internally consistent group of relational statements (concepts, definitions and propositions) that present a systematic view about a phenomenon and which is useful for description, explanation, prediction and control" (Bodie and Chitty, 1993).
>
> Nursing theories are used to describe, develop, disseminate, and use present knowledge in nursing. Nursing theories provide a framework for nurses to systematize their nursing actions: what to ask, what to observe, what to focus on, and what to think about. They provide a framework to develop new and validate current knowledge. They help to describe, explain, predict, and prescribe.
>
> Nursing theory is also used to: define commonalities of the variables in a stated field of inquiry; guide nursing research and actions; predict practice outcomes; and predict client response.

Theories can also be analyzed by type. In nursing, there are four types of theories: needs, interaction, outcome, and humanistic. Which theories apply to complex systems? A list of grand nursing theories and philosophies is located in the Appendix at the end of this chapter.

The Theory of Nursing Knowledge and Nursing Practice

Summary papers both accept and caution the use of complex thinking in nursing practice. Lela M. Holden (2005) concludes in her paper titled "Complex Adaptive Systems: Concept Analysis" that "the use of complex adaptive systems as a framework is increasing for a wide range of scientific applications, including nursing and health care management research. When nursing and other health care managers focus on increasing connections, diversity, and interactions, they increase information flow and promote creative adaptation referred to as self-organization. Complexity science builds on the rich tradition in nursing that views patients and nursing care from a systems perspective." (p. 651)

John Paley (2007), in the abstract for his paper "Complex Adaptive Systems and Nursing," warns against irrational application of complexity science in the nursing domain:

> There have been numerous references to complexity theory and complex systems in the recent healthcare literature, including nursing. However, exaggerated claims have (in my view) been made about how they can be applied to health service delivery, and there is a widespread tendency to misunderstand some of the concepts associated with complexity thinking (usually justified by describing the misconception as a metaphor). These concepts can be extended to systems and structures in healthcare organizations but, at this stage in the development of complexity science, only in a modest and very cautious way. In this paper I first outline some of the key ideas in the theory of complex adaptive systems, and then suggest that they have been distorted by a series of influential articles in the medical literature. I go on to present a simple case study of my own and undertake a complexity analysis of it. In the conclusion I suggest that we should beware of some outdated ideas being trotted out in the guise of complexity—an exciting and diverse area of enquiry that those old ideas do not, in fact, resemble. (p. 233)

Complexity science has advanced but remains a newer discipline than nursing science and practice. The application of all nursing theories highlighted in the previous section to complexity science cannot be covered in this chapter. But we can use both scientific theories to improve nursing care by starting with a simple evidenced-based approach to use data for simulation of existing conditions and test what-if scenarios to find the best approach within a system.

Finally, it is important to recognize the work of Betty Neuman, PhD, RN:

> Neuman's model is just that—a model, not a full theory. It is a conceptual framework, a visual representation, for thinking about humans and nurses and their interactions. The model views the person as a layered, multidimensional whole that is in constant dynamic interaction with the environment. The layers represent various levels of defense protecting the core being. The two major components in the model are stress reactions and systemic feedback loops. [The] client reacts to stress with lines of defense and resistance (Neuman, 1995). Continuous feedback loops fine-tune the lines of defense and resistance so as to achieve maximal level of stability. The client is in continuous and dynamic interaction with the environment. The exchanges between the environment and the client are reciprocal (each one is influenced by the other). The goal is to achieve optimal system stability and balance. Prevention is the main nursing intervention to achieve this balance. Primary, secondary, and tertiary prevention activities are used to attain, retain, and maintain system balance (George, 1996). (Heyman and Wolfe, 2000, "In Short")
>
> The main criticism of Neuman's Systems Model is that many of the concepts are not adequately defined, especially the difference between interpersonal and extrapersonal stressors. It seems as though interpersonal stressors should be a subcategory or special case of extrapersonal stressors. The term reaction needs to be better defined as well as the terms knowns and commons. In the model's nursing process, assessment and intervention are assumed, but not explicit, thus allowing anyone else to usurp these functions. This point needs to be addressed; do assessment and intervention belong to nursing, or can they be delegated to another profession? Finally, the question must be asked as to how accurate the model is in representing human beings and their interactions with the environment. While it is useful to think of people as layered and made up of five principles, it is not always easy to predict or describe their interplay. Moreover, since each layer is composed of all the person variables, it is not always clear as to what layer is being assessed in any operationalized variable. Despite the criticisms, the Neuman Systems Model is an excellent way for nurses and other health professionals to think about stress and prevention. (Heyman and Wolfe, 2000, "Criticisms")

In many respects this model brings us closer to the complexity science that started this discussion. Yet the evidence necessary to build a model and the choice of a modeling approach is not clearly delineated.

The next section discusses simulation modeling approaches, starting with an overview of the science and the toolsets used to create models.

Improvement Tools: Simulation Modeling

Simulation Modeling: What It Is, and How It Applies to the Nurse's Role in the CAS of the ED

Simulation modeling is a new frontier for most managers, providers, and architects working in the health care industry. Although successfully utilized in other industries, it has been slow to gain acceptance as a tool for health care process improvement, patient flow, and capacity planning and design.

In the pinnacle report from the Institute for Medicine, *Building a Better Delivery System: A New Engineering/Health Care Partnership*, Reid et al. (2005) discuss the use of systems engineering tools

> which have been used in a wide variety of applications to achieve major improvements in the quality, efficiency, safety, and/or customer-centeredness of processes, products, and services in a wide range of manufacturing and services industries. The health care sector as a whole has been very slow to embrace them, however, even though they have been shown to yield valuable returns to the small but growing number of health care organizations and clinicians that have applied them. (p. 2)

Barriers for utilizing simulation modeling within the three distinct but unified entities—health care, architecture, and simulation engineering—have limited its standardization as both a tool and a trusted resource.

> Statistical process controls, queuing theory, quality function deployment, failure-mode effects analysis, modeling and simulation, and human-factors engineering have been adapted to applications in health care delivery and used tactically by clinicians, care teams, and administrators in large health care organizations to improve the performance of discrete care processes, units, and departments. However, the strategic use of these and more information technology-intensive tools from the fields of enterprise and supply-chain management, financial engineering and risk analysis, and knowledge discovery in databases has been limited. With some adaptations, these tools could be used to measure, characterize, and optimize performance at higher levels of the health care system (e.g., individual health care organizations, regional care systems, the public health system, the health research enterprise, etc.). The most promising systems-engineering tools and areas of associated research identified by the committee are listed in [Table 6.1]. (Reid et al. (2005, 2–3)

Table 6.1 Systems Engineering Tools and Research for Health Care Delivery

Tools/Research Areas	Levels of Application			
	Patient	Team	Organization	Environment
Systems-Design Tools				
Concurrent engineering and quality function		X	X	
Human-factors tools	X	X	X	X
Failure mode effects analysis		X	X	
Systems-Analysis Tools				
Modeling and Simulation				
Queuing methods	X	X	X	
Discrete-event simulation	X	X	X	X
Enterprise-Management Tools				
Supply-chain management		X	X	X
Game theory and contracts		X	X	X
Systems-dynamics models		X	X	X
Productivity measuring and monitoring		X	X	X
Financial Engineering and Risk Analysis Tools				
Stochastic analysis			X	X
Value-at-risk			X	X
Optimization tools for individual decision making		X	X	X
Distributed decision making: market models and agency theory			X	X
Knowledge Discovery in Databases				
Data mining			X	X
Predictive modeling		X	X	X
Neural networks		X	X	X
Systems-Control Tools				
Statistical process control	X	X	X	
Scheduling		X	X	

Note: Italics indicate areas with significant research opportunities.

Understanding the Tools

We recognize there are a vast number of modeling approaches and tools designed to assist the health care client in understanding their existing state and predicting improvements on that state.

Dr. Terry Young has demonstrated that finding the right tool is about being fully aware of all the tools that can be used. Through the RIGHT (Research Into Global Healthcare Tools) project his team of academicians has created a handbook titled *Modeling and Simulation Techniques for Supporting Healthcare Decision Making: A Selection Framework* (www.right.org.uk) for identifying several variables in choosing the right tool. The O'Hara HealthCare Consultants LLC (OHC) team basic toolset includes representative models as identified in Table 6.2.

To offer an alternative explanation of the OHC toolset approach, we have created a simple scenario-based questionnaire to offer beginning health care managers a starting point to determine which modeling approach best meets their needs. This is clearly not an all inclusive list and, it could be argued, it actually is quite limiting. However, it is my experience that a simplistic, scenario-based approach is most effective in helping the new or novice modeling champion understand this very complicated technology. It also helps the model champion to explain it to their decisions makers. During the discussion, the customer can begin to identify with some portion of these five scenarios and can also begin to see the value of simulation modeling tools. Furthermore, the customer starts to recognize ways in which scenarios (or charges from stakeholders) have impacted the desire to use simulation modeling, as well as how any combination of these approaches can be helpful. This questionnaire was developed with Jim Walsh,

Table 6.2   The OHC Basic Toolset

Model Type	OHC Tool	Description
Discrete event simulation (DES) or process model	EXTENDSIM	Efficient, graphical programming tool; EXTENSIVE Experience
Bayesian belief network	NETICA	Algorithm learns relationships among data; uses diverse data sources; behavior model basis; conditional statistical models; team has integrated with EXTENDSIM
Optimization	CPLEX (Others)	Integer Programming and Other Optimization tools can be Integrated with Process/ABM
Agent-based model	HEAT	HEAT (Healthcare Efficacy and Architectural Analysis Tool) is a team proprietary, health care specific agent-based model; represents agent interaction and adaptation to processes, architecture, and technologies created with SPARTA Inc.

SPARTA Inc., and Mark Sullivan, Mark Sullivan Architects. Although it has a facility-based focus, it has been tested with operations mangers.

MODELING QUESTIONS, APPROACH, AND VALUE ADDED PERSPECTIVE TO HELP DETERMINE A MODELING PROJECT PLAN

1. Patient Volume Predictions (an ED)
    a. Questions answered: What is the projected patient volume? How do I know how many beds or employees to plan for in new design?
    b. Approach: Influence diagrams, Bayesian belief networks
    c. Value added: Builds on existing methods; provides efficient means to model data; provides distribution around projections
2. Facility Capacity and Sizing Estimates
    a. Questions answered: What are the facility top-level requirements that best meet performance metrics: capacities of key resources (waiting areas, beds, etc)?
    b. Approach: Apply statistical methods, queuing theory, and discrete event simulation
    c. Value added:
        i. Right sizing of facility and key resources reduces risk and saves on facility costs; provides design team with enhanced information for more efficient and effective design process
        ii. Provides planners with tools for quick what-ifs on key design parameters
        iii. Accurate design requirements lead to cost savings and reduced risk
3. Early Assessment and Visualization of the Design (an ED)
    a. Questions answered: What designs best meet overall performance goals? What are the critical design challenges and what are the alternative and best solutions?
    b. Approach: Apply agent-based modeling to assess facility utilization; apply visualization techniques
    c. Value added:
        i. Facilitates design team coordination and insights into potential problems; allows consideration of alternative designs in a "virtual" way, making process more efficient and less costly
        ii. Provides "virtual" tool to examine alternative designs
        iii. Efficient means to arrive at well thought-out solutions

4. Early Integration of Processes, Technologies into New Facility (ED and relationship to adjacencies)
   a. Questions answered: How do current and projected processes and technologies integrate into the facility design? What are the integration challenges and solutions?
   b. Approach: Agent-based modeling allows simulation of how processes and technologies will perform in a specific layout
   c. Value added:
      i. Provides correct total system view for the customer; reduces risks and leads to cost savings
      ii. Adds value through insight into integration of processes and technology with facility
      iii. Ability to prepare for new facility start up; effective use day one
      iv. Use as an orientation tool to help users "work" in the new space before and during the construction process.
5. Total Hospital Analyses (ED within whole hospital and competition for resources)
   a. Questions answered: What are the key points of interoperability between the departments? How does the design facilitate physical and informational interoperability?
   b. Approach: Agent-based model and discrete event simulation allows assessment of department interactions and view of hospital as a total design
   c. Value added:
      i. Cost savings from total system balancing; more efficient design process and convergence; early identification and resolution of issues
      ii. Ability to provide system of systems insight; is value added to the customer?
      iii. More efficient design process and convergence
      iv. Early identification and resolution of issues
      v. Excellent way to have health care systems view to determine reuse, demolition, merging, and new catchment area utilization

Although the data requirements vary with each of the five modeling approaches, our systems thinking philosophy remains unchanged. Another viewpoint is represented in Table 6.3 by Walsh, our simulation engineer.

Table 6.3 A Needs-Based Table with Rationale

Need	Applicable Model Type	Rationale
Resource capacity analysis	Discrete event simulation (DES) or process model	Focus is on queues and utilization
Process assessment, enhancement	DES or process model, agent-based model (ABM)	First order is process model; ABM addresses behavior complexities and interactions
Scheduling approach optimization	DES or process model, optimization tools (integer programming)	Scheduling is a resource allocation problem
Decide, prepare for new technology	DES or process model, ABM	ABM represents how behavior adapts to new technology
Layout optimization	ABM, distance minimization	First order can be optimization; ABM represents interactive behavior with space
Staff selection, training criteria	Bayesian belief network (BBN)	BBN can discover complex influences on performance
Quality/safety influences and indicators; benchmarks, standards, guidelines	ABM, BBN	ABM represents behavior; BBN can point to behaviors that correlate to quality/safety issues

Understanding the Simulation Project

The first step in a modeling project is to understand the questions you would like answered. As we discussed in the previous section, there are several ways to frame the question, issue, or hypothesis. Modeling requirements cannot be established without this foundation of questions. It can be framed as a set of intuitive or gut feelings, such as "If we extend our hours of operation, we can see more patients and decrease length of stay in waiting room." As an alternative, try writing a theory or hypothesis to disprove this, such as "Any additional treatment rooms in our emergency department will not improve patient flow; however adding an admission discharge transfer (ADT) nurse will." Once you have written the question, theory, or hypothesis you are ready to begin dialogue with your modeling and simulation engineer. Often a facility or health care system has purchased a software package that it believes is multipurpose and may even solve all its modeling needs. This it not always going to be the case.

It is important to establish an interactive approach with the engineers. They may, from their experience, see other alternatives that you have not thought of or software you have not purchased. Finally, you will be ready to start down a path. Be prepared to uncover the possibility that the modeling approach you have agreed upon might change. The rationale should be explained clearly enough so one can make an informed decision on value-added benefits, time, and cost to project.

The majority of health care simulation models are discrete event simulation (DES) models, also known as process models. This is noted in a literature search of simulation modeling of emergency departments. However, more recently health care modeling has moved toward agent-based models. Smith and Feied (1999) describe the emergency department as a "complex system" but do not mention a modeling approach. Other authors have begun to describe alternative modeling approaches. In the paper "Computer Terminal Placement and Workflow in an Emergency Department: An Agent-Based Model," Poynton et al. (2007) modeled a hypothetical ED to discover the effect of location of electronic medical record with computer physician order entry on patient outcome. In this model agents are the patients, the providers, and the computer terminals. Results showed bedside terminals more efficient than clustered terminals, but the authors comment that the low fidelity of this study necessitates further research. The work of Laskowski and Mukhi (2009) is a combination of hypothetical and actual research, and describes efforts for integrating multiple emergency departments and the diversion protocols. A few other papers exist on this specific modeling approach and can be searched by the reader.

Next, I will discuss briefly a very simple way of understanding the differences between the process model and the agent-based model, as illustrated in Figure 6.2.

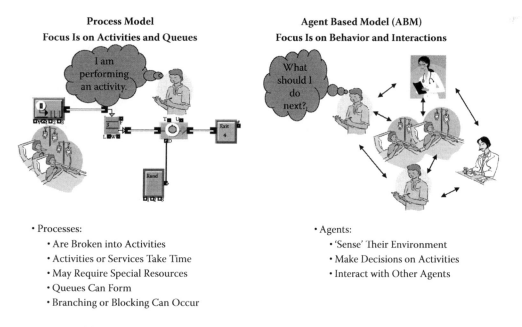

Process Model	Agent Based Model (ABM)
Focus Is on Activities and Queues	**Focus Is on Behavior and Interactions**

- Processes:
  - Are Broken into Activities
  - Activities or Services Take Time
  - May Require Special Resources
  - Queues Can Form
  - Branching or Blocking Can Occur

- Agents:
  - 'Sense' Their Environment
  - Make Decisions on Activities
  - Interact with Other Agents

- *Process Models Are Effective Means to Study Processes and Resource Utilization*
- *As Processes, Interactions and Number of Actors Increase, ABM Modeling Is Effective Approach*

Figure 6.2   (Courtesy of Jim Walsh, SPARTA Inc.)

Once the model type has been determined by the management team with the engineering team, it is critical to plan the model building process. I would like to propose an outside-the-box first step in planning your project by reading Law's "pitfalls to the successful completion of a simulation study" (2006, 77–78):

■ Failure to have a well-defined set of objectives at the beginning of the simulation study
■ Failure to have the entire project team involved at the beginning of the study
■ Inappropriate level of model detail
■ Failure to communicate with management throughout the course of the simulation study
■ Misunderstanding of simulation by management
■ Treating a simulation study as if it were primarily an exercise in computer programming
■ Failure to have people with knowledge of simulation methodology and statistics on the modeling team
■ Failure to collect good system data (refer to data collection system)
■ Inappropriate simulation software
■ Obliviously using simulation-software packages, whose complex macro statements may not be well documented and may not implement the desired modeling logic
■ Belief that easy-to-use simulation packages, which require little or no programming, require a significantly lower level of technical competence
■ Misuse of animation
■ Failure to account correctly for sources of randomness in the actual system
■ Using arbitrary distributions (e.g., normal, uniform, or triangular as input to the simulation
■ Analyzing the output data from one simulation run (replications) using formulas that assume independence
■ Making a single replication of a particular system design and treating the output statistics as the "true answers"
■ Failure to have a warm-up period, if the steady-state behavior of a system is of interest
■ Comparing alternative system designs on the basis of one replication of each design
■ Using the wrong performance measures

Steps to Plan a Model

A simple model plan should include the following, as described by Law (2006, 67). Law cautions that these steps are not simply part of a sequential process but may require returning to previous steps.

1. Formulate the problem and plan the study
2. Collect data and define a model
3. Assumptions in the document are valid? If no return to step 2; if yes, proceed to step 4
*4. Construct a computer program and verify
*5. Make pilot runs
*6. Programmed model valid? If no return to step 2; if yes proceed to step 7
**7. Design experiments
8. Make production runs
9. Analyze output data
10. Document, present, and use results
  * Steps 4 through 6 are iterative.
  ** The Design of Experiments stage requires an understanding of factors (variables) and levels (range of data measures).

In summary, it is important to start out with a simple model that "runs."

The OHC team developed a *model scoping* questionnaire to help determine project parameters. The core tenants of the questionnaire are:

1. Goals
2. Patient profiling and the health care program
3. Processes or procedures
4. Facilities (applies to departments, networks, communities)
5. Resources: Human and equipment
6. Revenue and costs
7. Model accuracy
8. Animation requirements
9. Reporting requirements
10. Training requirements
11. Project time envelope
12. Project budget envelope

The initial model should be running before you add complexity to the model and time to the project.

Data (Clinical, Operational, Architectural)

To build a health care simulation model it is necessary to understand the health care unit (for instance, the ED) as part of a whole system and not as a single entity. This does not mean that the modeler will be able to incorporate all of the relational items into this OHC systems flow model. However, it is recommended that the nurse model champion have a complete understanding of all of the components described next. (I recognize and fully appreciate other health care workers' value as support or as sole model champions. However, it is this author's perspective that nurses have a unique and global understanding of daily operations, patient care, and space utilization that I believe makes them ideal model champions.) Not only does this prevent misunderstandings about the system being modeled, but it provides a framework for data collection and what-if scenario building (design of experiments).

Start your master data set by following the OHC Systems Compass (Figure 6.3) beginning with the mission statements of the health care system, facility, and department. Evaluate the voice of the customer (VOC) data (surveys, complaints, satisfactions reports). Include the relationship to internal patient flow initiatives and benchmarks. Place the unit of study within the adjacent (philosophically and architecturally) internal units such as staffing, IS (information systems), IT (information technology), safety, and so forth. Finally, examine supporting data, benchmarks, guidelines, and laws related to the unit being modeled at the clinical program, department, health care facility, network, community, and state and federal or public health level.

Often this master data set nursing activity is done in conjunction with the process flow mapping or creation of the influence diagram. Since this book includes an excellent discussion on how to accomplish process mapping (see Chapter 2), I will not detail it here. I do offer an alternative starting point (especially if a Bayesian network model is used (Figure 6.4)), and that is the influence diagram (Figures 6.5 and 6.6).

Data collection at each point on this OHC systems compass will be both qualitative and quantitative. It is critical to work with the performance improvement engineers or statistical personnel at your facility to provide a unified way to create the master database. Do not proceed down a blind path. Based on experience I recommend starting with a one-month data set. This can then be used by the modelers to build the model processes. While this is being crafted, go back and collect either a six-month or twelve-month data set (depending on project time and budget envelopes).

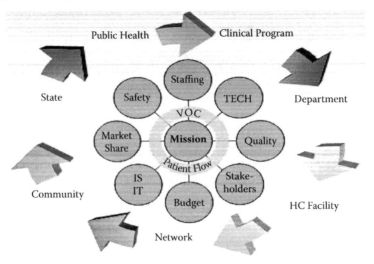

Figure 6.3   Whole systems diagram.

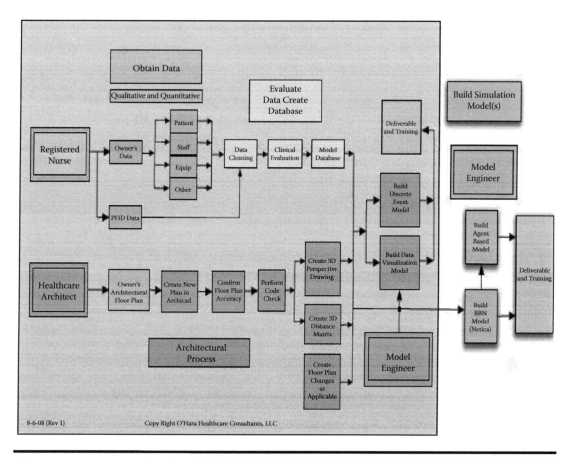

Figure 6.4   An example of a simulation modeling process. (Source: O'Hara HealthCare Consultants, LLC.)

Much of the initial time dedicated to a modeling project is simply locating the data resources within the facility. Do not underestimate the value and enormity of this task. If this is not your full-time job (and most likely it is not) allow for three times the amount of hours you anticipate it will take. Alternatively, ensure that the project has allocated this activity to either the modeling team or a dedicated person at your facility.

It is critical to put the data in context of the clinical program you are studying. Look beneath the data at the underlying patient population characteristics. Also, be aware of "special causes" or outliers. Despite their rarity or minimal probability in a data set, they may create a different process or bottleneck that requires contingency planning. The OHC systems approach to health care simulation and modeling brings together three key processes: clinical, architecture, and engineering. Figure 6.4 provides an overview of the data collection steps related to the nursing and architectural existing conditions. The traditional validation, verification, and accreditation steps of the engineering process are assumed in the "Build" steps.

Influence diagrams help nurses to apply systems thinking, starting at the bottom (unit level) and working up or at the top-down level. These diagrams are

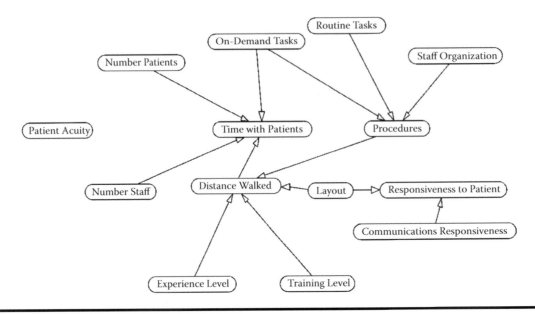

Figure 6.5 Example of influence diagram of nurse performance metrics and factors. Initial focus: define the influences/factors, define the performance metrics and the relationship between them. (Source: O'Hara HealthCare Consultants, LLC.)

simple to draw and do not require software. However, if a Bayesian network is utilized, then software such as Netica (Norysis) is helpful to creating the influence diagrams.

The following examples were created by our project engineer, Jim Walsh, (Figure 6.5 and Figure 6.6). They demonstrate micro- and macro-level thinking and can be done by the nursing model champion.

The data collection process provides the modeling team and customer the opportunity to identify and point out all processes, but especially those that are broken. At this point, I recommend the customer be notified of such a process for two reasons: 1. if possible, stop or change the process if patient care is at risk or could be improved, and 2. to discuss whether or not to exclude this process from the model. Finally it is important to keep a log or chart of special causes, outliers, and data sources.

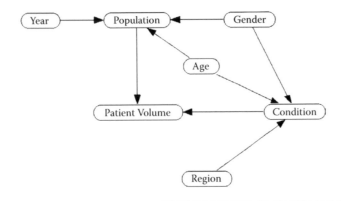

Figure 6.6 Example of influence diagram of patient volume projection. (Source: O'Hara HealthCare Consultants, LLC.)

Scope and What-Ifs

Design of Experiments

Once the scope of the model has been established, it is important to design the experiments. It helps to divide the overall experiment into the work environment (architecture), the workforce and operations (engineering), and the clinical processes (flow and clinical benchmarks) experiments, using these three domains as a guide. From each of these disciplines, the team should identify factors which drive the performance and can be modeled to demonstrate a change.

Once the clinical team has created a list of scenarios to be tested (using a hypothesis, flow map, or architectural case study matrix) the list must be reviewed with the engineers. A great deal of disappointment can occur if this phase of the modeling process is not fully vetted. Furthermore, the engineers need to be able to quantify the experiments and code them in the model structures.

The what-if scenarios should be designed after a review of other existing models in the facility, other national models of the same clinical entity, and national data to use for benchmarking.

Working with Engineers

Simulation modeling engineers are experts in their field. They may or may not have an understanding of the health care setting they are modeling. It is the job and duty of the nurse model champion to make sure the engineers understand the clinical area under study. This includes a data inventory as well as taking the time to initiate process flow or value stream maps. Software is not needed for this effort. Simply drawing on paper your perception of the flow in the area of study is the best way to know your domain. If you cannot explain your department to your own health care setting's peers recognizing their multiple viewpoints, it will be difficult to explain it to the engineers. I have worked on projects gathering and collecting this qualitative and quantitative data in a way that has actually been revealing to the entire in-house team. As one nurse leader said, "You know our departments better than we do!" That was not strictly the case; it was that I was able to understand the cross-functional utilization of the departments' staff, space, and patients in a bird's-eye view: one that is objective and without judgment.

Simulation modeling is what I call the "great equalizer." There is no department better, stronger, or able to leap tall buildings than another. Often user groups see one another from a completely different perspective when sitting down to objectively discuss resource flow, process, and operations. The never ending hunt to find secret and unused spaces tucked away in a hospital can be ended if everyone understands the whole picture of how resources and space are utilized, and affect the whole hospital. If you can explain your department operations to other professionals (architects and modeling engineers), you may gain insight into your own processes. Even more important, however, is you will see how each domain is intrinsically and critically linked: All professionals effect patient care change.

At the early model scoping phase in which schedule planning occurs, include time (calendar and budget) for review meetings. Be sure to meet your data collection, model review, and other deadlines so as not to hold up the engineers' process and schedule.

I cannot recommend strongly enough the importance of taking the time to learn about modeling. The more you understand, the better you will be able to provide the right information at the right time. Furthermore, you have a responsibility to your stakeholders to teach them about your model. Engineers build and deliver models for various reasons. Some models are built without data because the owner of the data does not want or cannot release the data. Some models are built for analysis purposes where the engineer will receive data and input it into the model and provide analysis for the customer. In this case the customer is not interested in owning the model. Other deliverables include a combination of all the cases in which the customer hires the engineer to build the model, populate it with data, run the model, and analyze the model output. Often this case includes client/customer training on running the model and creating scenarios and analyzing results.

When engaging an engineering team, ask them what they are used to delivering. This will also help you to understand the licensing and ownership questions. Although these are important issues, they are not part of this chapter.

Do not be afraid to discuss the model databases or the techniques employed to create the model. Remember that this is a collaborative approach and in each stage, testing the model will help determine direction and uncover results that may not have been discovered. In order to be respectful of all time constraints, identify your interests up front at the model scoping phase. Additional meetings may increase the cost of the project and if not determined early can lead to disappointment and a sense of failing to meet expectations.

If after establishing the working approach the engineers do not share their status, call a timeout and meet to reestablish team goals. Everyone should be free to question the modeling process. It is important to identify tasks and responsibilities early in the process. If you are not responsible for building the model, do not try to write the code for it. By respecting the professional disciplines, both engineers and nurses and other health care professionals can create a synergistic and dynamic modeling process and deliver a successful simulation modeling project.

Putting It All Together (Using an ED Case Study)

Keep in mind that nurses are key agents within the complex adaptive systems of the hospital and more specifically for this case study in the ED. The work on this model was created by Robin Clark of QMT group, Henry Bell formerly of Smoky Mountain Simulation Services, and Mark Sullivan of Mark Sullivan Architects. In this systems process modeling approach we incorporated system thinking but designed the model as a process model.

Table 6.4   Distance Matrix

LOCATION	Walk-In Entrance	Registration	Waiting Room	Registration Interview L	Registration Interview R	Triage 1	Triage 2	Consult	Lab	Ambulance Parking	Trauma A	Trauma B
Walk-In Entrance	0	94'	39'	55'	50'	63'	74'	79'	78'	238'	199'	199'
Registration	94'	0	109'	52'	58'	24'	38'	43'	48'	178'	138'	138'
Waiting Room	39'	109'	0	70'	65'	37'	47'	53'	93'	253'	213'	213'
Registration Interview L	55'	52'	70'	0	14'	48'	56'	62'	36'	196'	157'	157'
Registration Interview R	50'	58'	65'	14'	0	53'	62'	67'	41'	201'	162'	162'
Triage 1	63'	24'	37'	48'	53'	0	32'	37'	44'	171'	132'	132'
Triage 2	74'	38'	47'	56'	62'	32'	0	26'	53'	161'	121'	121'
Consult	79'	43'	53'	62'	67'	37'	26'	0	55'	158'	119'	119'
Lab	78'	48'	93'	36'	41'	44'	53'	55'	0'	189'	150'	150'
Ambulance Parking	238'	178'	253'	196'	201'	171'	161'	158'	189'	0	92'	92'
Trauma A	199'	138'	213'	157'	162'	132'	121'	119'	150'	92'	0	31'
Trauma B	199'	138'	213'	157'	162'	132'	121'	119'	150'	92'	31'	0
RN Station 1	81'	51'	96'	39'	44'	46'	55'	58'	32'	152'	112'	112'

Source: Excerpt courtesy of MSA.

We have used whole system thinking in our practice. The architectural database (Table 6.4) in this ED case study includes the distance matrix and other travel distances (Table 6.5) related to ED access and travel paths (Figure 6.7).

This case study demonstrates the following components:

1. Purpose of model
2. Model layout
3. Database
4. Animation
5. Notebook
6. Experiments

Assumptions were made that individual nurses' walking speed was not considered in system performance.

Table 6.5   Other Travel Distances Related to ED Access and Travel Paths: All ED Locations to All Main Hospital Locations

	Emergency/Observation					Diagnostic Center
Level	1st Floor	1st Floor	1st Floor	1st Floor	1st Floor	1st Floor
Location	Chest Observation 1365	Chest Observation 1366	Chest Observation 1367	Isolation 1380	Isolation 1382	Diagnostic Imaging Front Door
ED Back Door	39′	44′	61′	70′	87′	45′
ED Trauma						

Source: Excerpt courtesy of MSA.

Note: Measurements are from back door of ED to front door of each room/department. Measurements do not include the vertical distance traveled on the elevator.

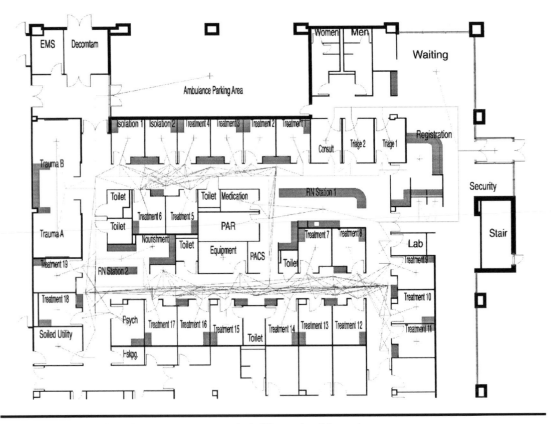

Figure 6.7   Travel paths. (Courtesy Mark Sullivan Architects)

Purpose of Model

The purpose of model is twofold: (1) experiment with capacity of waiting room and capacity of treatment rooms and (2) test performance measures such as utilization of treatment rooms and length of patient stay.

Model Layout

Figure 6.8 shows the model layout.

1. Buttons for Database, Microsoft Access Output Reports, Access, Experiment Manager
2. Slider for patient volume
3. Cloned parameters for beds in use, waiting room seats in use, waiting room seats available, observation/chest pain seats, RNs (registered nurses)
4. Hierarchical blocks for patient arrivals, waiting room, patient triage, patient treatment, patient lab/testing, patient observation, CP center, patient disposition
5. Patient icon legend

The patient arrivals construct (Figure 6.9) generates the patients entering the model.

The waiting room construct (Figure 6.10) models the waiting room. This includes the waiting room from sign-in to triage as well as a temporary holding area after triage if there is no treatment room available.

The patient triage construct (Figure 6.11) models the triage logic. After triage, the patients will either go to a treatment room, go back to the waiting room, or elope.

The patient treatment construct (Figure 6.12) models the usage of the treatment rooms.

The patient lab/testing construct (Figure 6.13) models the additional delay time of lab and radiology.

The patient observation construct (Figure 6.14) models the usage of the observation beds.

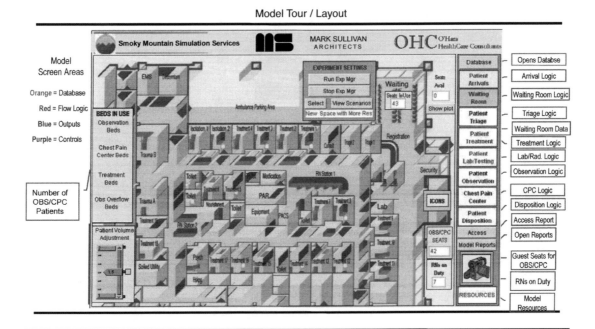

Figure 6.8   Emergency Department Model Main Screen.

Model Tour / Layout - Arrivals

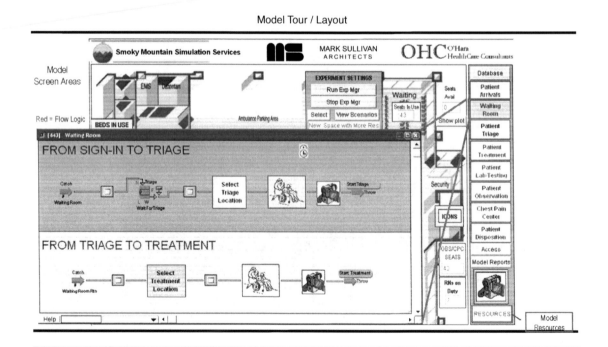

Figure 6.9   Patient arrivals.

The patient disposition construct (Figure 6.15) models the disposition of the patients. From here the patients will find the visitors they brought with them and leave.

The resources construct (Figure 6.16) models the usage of resources in the model. This includes treatment rooms, isolation beds, psych beds, trauma beds,

Model Tour / Layout

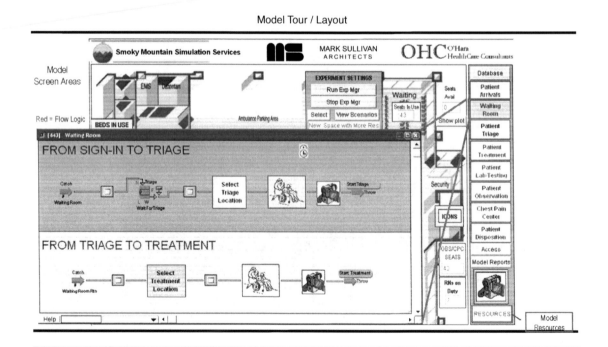

Figure 6.10   Waiting room.

Model Tour / Layout

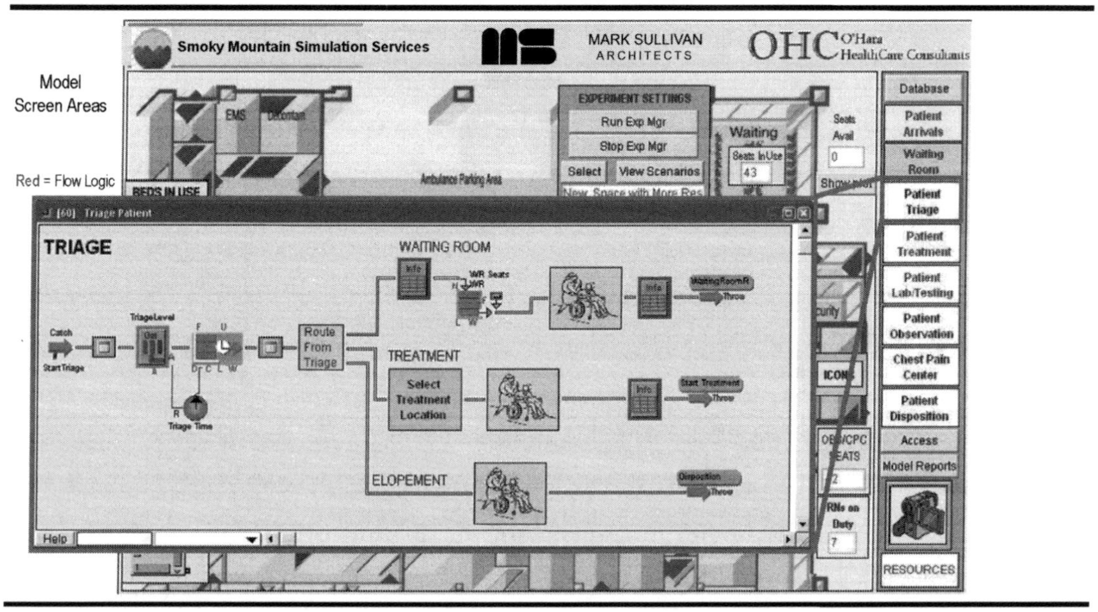

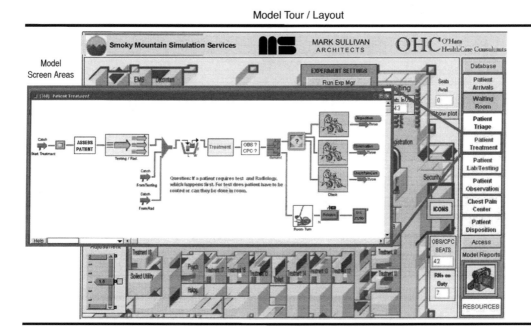

Figure 6.11 Patient triage.

observation beds, chest pain beds, triage, waiting room seats, clerks, RNs, MDs, liaisons, and ambulances.

The Microsoft Access button (Figure 6.17) launches access to the case history data and reports can be generated from it.

The model report button opens (Figure 6.18) the model notebook. The model notebook displays the important performance measures of the model output.

Model Tour / Layout

Figure 6.12 Patient treatment.

Model Tour / Layout

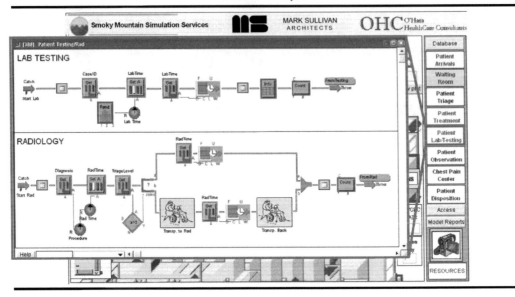

Figure 6.13   Patient lab/testing.

Ancillary Services are modeled to determine time, distance and processes
(to mention a few variables/factors). It is helpful when deciding on physically
locating internal satellite labs and services within the department or to use main
hospital services.

Model Tour / Layout

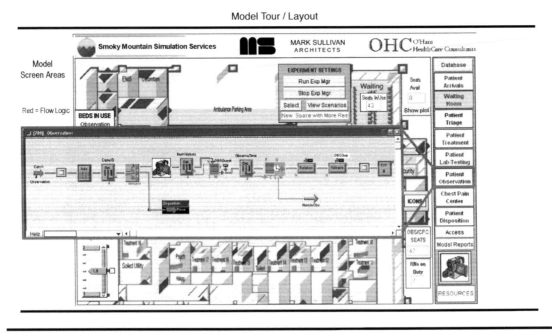

Figure 6.14   Patient observation.

Patient Observation modeling may require an additional companion model if
the unit is a separate cost center with a different staff. Adjacency does not mean
that Observation or Chest Pain Centers are all part of the primary emergency
services cost center.

Model Tour / Layout

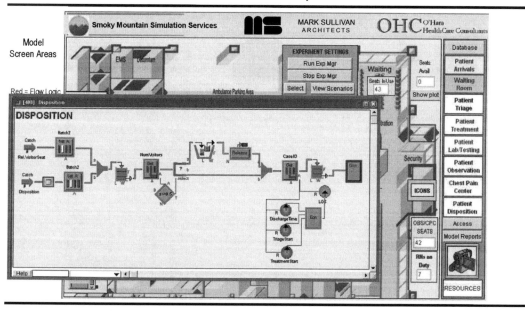

Figure 6.15 Patient disposition.

Model Tour / Layout

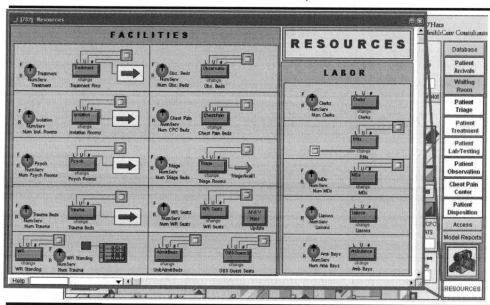

Figure 6.16 Resources.

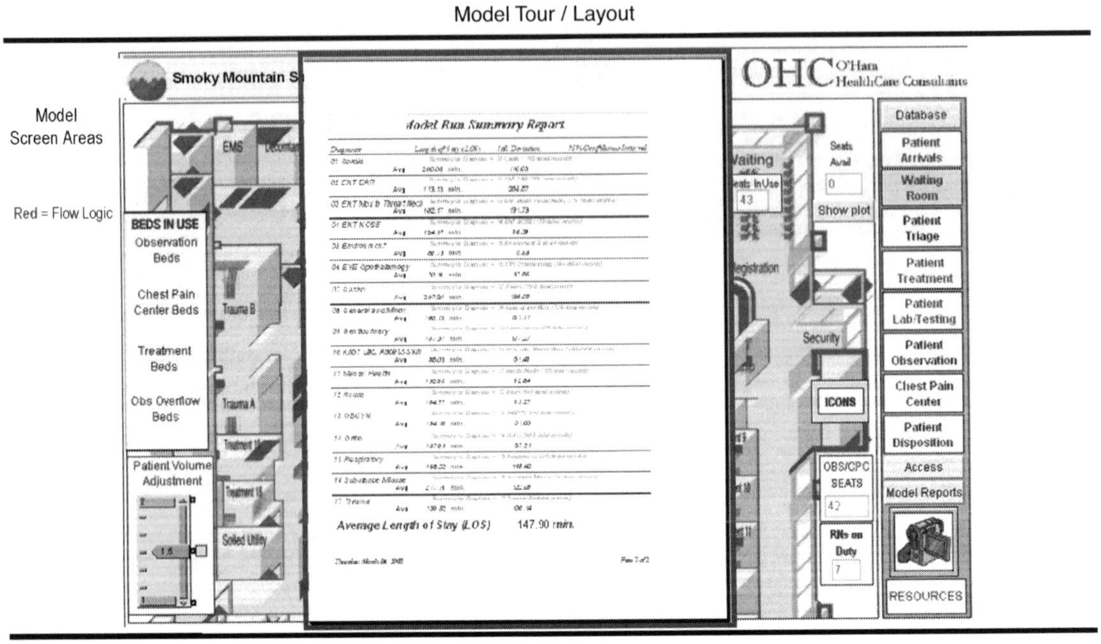

Model Tour / Layout

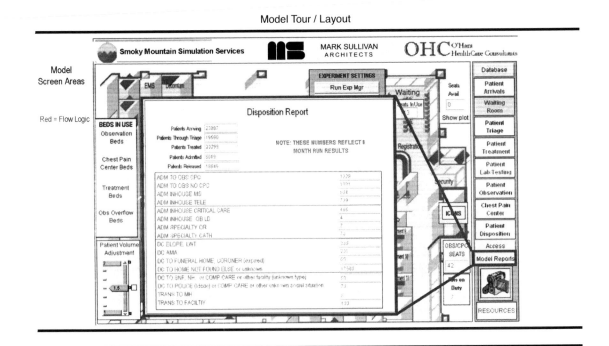

Figure 6.17   Microsoft Access Reports are viewed with a click on the "Access" button.

Model Tour / Layout

Figure 6.18   Model report button.

Database

The model database (Figure 6.19) is used for mostly every parameter.

Input Tables (A)
- Arrival hour (throughout 24-hour day)
- Arrival statistics (patient arrivals)
- EKG procedure time
- General delay parameters
- General process delays
- Lab procedure time
- Location distance matrix
- Nurse schedule

Input Tables (B)
- Observation location probability data (based on diagnosis code)
- Patient probabilities
- Patient process times
- Radiology procedure times
- Resources
- Room turnover
- Triage levels (determine if triage system is diagnosis- or resource-based)
- Various probabilities

Model Database

- Used for Majority of Model Parameters
- Input Tables
- Detail/Log Table – Case History
- Input Tables Values Based on 12 Months of Data

SAMPLE INPUT TABLE

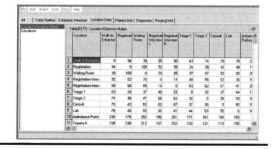

Figure 6.19   Model database.

Detail/Log Table - Case History

- One Record for Every Patient
- Describes the Detailed Patient Flow
- This table should be used for ...
  - Detailed Validation
  - Model Analysis

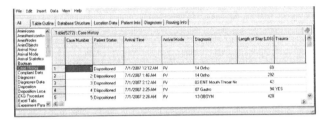

This is an example (but not exhaustive) of masked patient variables.

Figure 6.20   The fields in this table are based on questions you are trying to answer.

Input Tables (C)
  – Diagnosis (Dx) Data
    • Triage level
    • Probability of radiology
    • Radiology procedure probability
    • Probability of lab
    • Lab procedure probability
    • Probability of EKG
    • Probability of observation
    • Duration of observation
  – Diagnosis Data
    • Probability of chest pain center (CPC)
    • Duration of CPC
    • Probability of trauma
    • Probability isolation required
    • Disposition location
    • Triage to room time
    • Room-to-doctor (Dr) time
    • Dr-to-Dx time

Animation

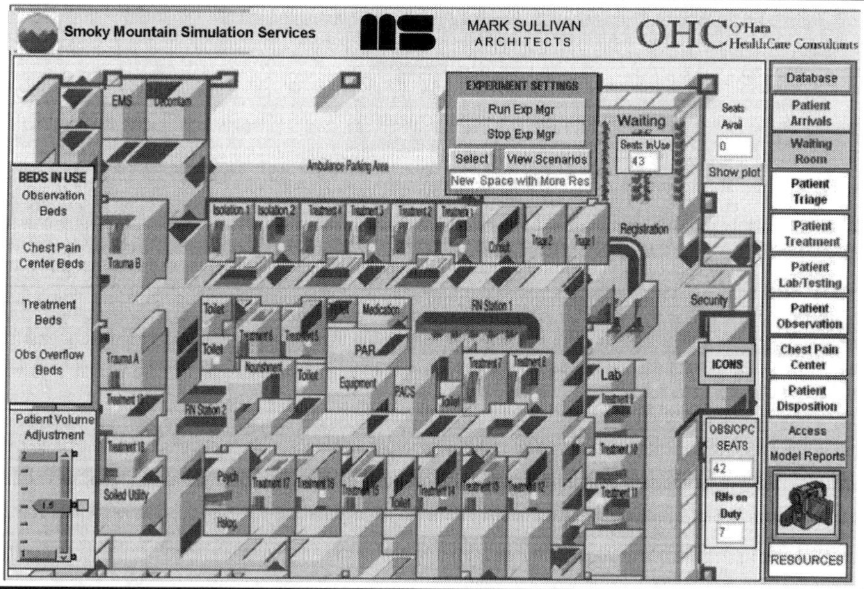

Figure 6.21   Animation movements of patients.

Animation

Figure 6.21 and Figure 6.22 show animation movements of patients using icon legends that represent the triage system.

Animation is not just "eye candy." Some team members learn by observing real data flowing through virtual floor plans. This is a value-added benefit that promotes multidisciplinary discussion and thoughtful "what-if" scenario planning.

Notebook (Figure 6.23)

- Control panel for experiment manager
- Disposition report
- Resource usage plots
    - Treatment, isolation, psych (mental health)
    - Trauma, observation, chest pain center (CPC) bed, triage
    - Waiting room seats
    - Nurses, MDs
- Admit beds used

Animation

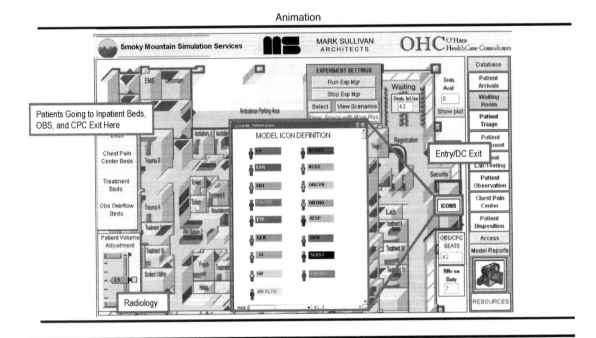

Figure 6.22 Animation movements of patients with icon legends.

Notebook

- Model Control Panel
- Disposition Report
- Resource Usage Plots

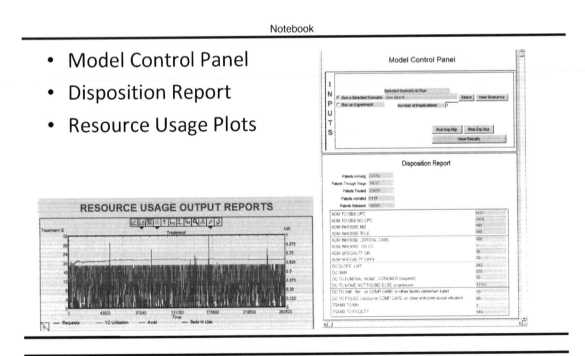

Figure 6.23 The Notebook is a fully customizable screen for running and reviewing simplified results.

Demand Factor

Demand Factor	Patients	Notes
80%	25,600	
90%	28,800	
100%	32,000	Current Volume
110%	35,200	
120%	38,400	
130%	41,600	Predicted in yr 2016
140%	44,800	
150%	48,000	
160%	51,200	
170%	54,400	

Figure 6.24 Demand factor in the illustrated example.

Experimentation

- Critical factors
  - The model was run to determine sensitivity to the critical factors.
  - The factors are manipulated to assess their impact on system performance.
- Performance measures
  - The performance measures were predetermined and identified in the model building stage to gauge system performance.
- In the illustrated example:
  - Factors
    - Demand: The demand factor (Figure 6.24) was varied from 80% current volume to 170% of current volume to determine the sensitivity to demand.
    - Treatment room capacity: The number of treatment rooms (Figure 6.25) varied from 17 to 23 rooms to show the sensitivity to capacity. All other rooms were left the same. Using four treatment room levels
      - 17 treatment rooms
      - 19 treatment rooms (proposed level)
      - 21 treatment rooms
      - 23 treatment rooms
  - Performance measures
    - Treatment room utilization (Figure 6.25)
    - Length of stay (Figure 6.26)
- Percent to waiting room first (Figure 6.27)

Experiments – Treatment Room Utilization

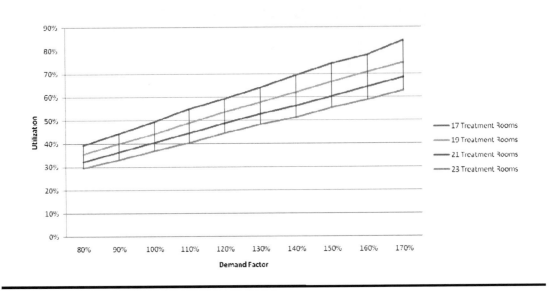

Figure 6.25 Number of treatment rooms in the illustrated example.

Experiments – Average Length of Stay

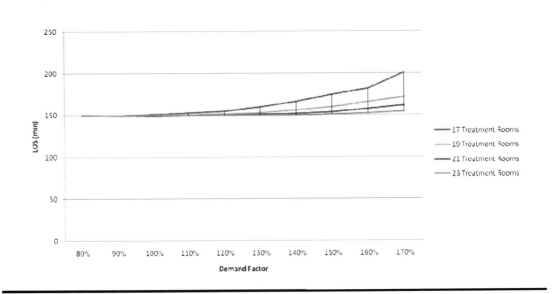

Figure 6.26 Average length of stay.

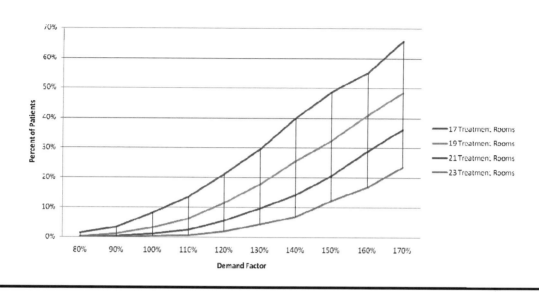

Figure 6.27   Percent to waiting room first.

Experience

My experience in simulation modeling has spanned five years and many models and engineers. The whole systems models we have delivered have been for cardiovascular systems (inpatient and outpatient electrophysiology labs, cardiac catheterization, and vascular labs); surgical systems including preadmission testing, pre- and postoperative day surgery care, and post anesthesia care unit (PACU), as well as a surgical suite with a block scheduling feature; and the emergency department. In the surgical model we incorporated construction phasing as well as cost of surgery and variance during phasing. Cost analyses should be incorporated into model structures and if it is not possible should be part of the cost-benefit analysis done using the model output.

Currently, we are completing our first agent-based model using nurse agents and starting our second model in which we use nurse and patient agents. Both models are for inpatient units and use radio frequency identification (RFID) technology.

Lessons Learned

The nursing perspective in a health care simulation modeling project is critical. I believe all health care modeling projects should be led by a nurse. However, that does not in any way change the equal importance of both the simulation engineers and the architect in fulfilling their professional obligations and objectives.

Understanding the project scope and the validation, verification, and perhaps the accreditation process are all part of this significant responsibility. If you do not understand what you can expect, make a point to clearly define your understanding.

Finally, simulation engineers offer a unique understanding of the world from which we and our patients can benefit. Find the right engineers for the project since you will be working with them for a concentrated period of time. Make sure their experience is as seriously considered as their ability to collaborate with you.

Ask to see a model run. Although an AVI file is quick and planned, be sure you can see how the engineers use the software so you have a very clear picture of their abilities and the ease of use with the software.

The analysis process should consist of dedicated time in face-to-face meetings. Although it is possible to receive the modeling results in an electronic meeting, nothing compares to the value created by sitting with the engineers and discovering emerging results, or finding a true improvement opportunity. But it is a give-and-take event; the time should be clearly allocated and uninterrupted, and therefore produce real value.

Future: Summary and Discussion

Not all software, processes, and engineers are alike, equal, or interchangeable. Answers are still needed to questions such as: What standards exist for simulation models and engineers? How can I determine if a model built in one software package has the same results as that built in another? What data collection process should I expect to be universal to simulation model building?

Too often we implement tools that work in one industry without truly understanding the commonalties and differences for application in the health care industry. This can be seen today as the health care industry makes efforts to implement new technology that "solves a problem" but adds more work, cost, or frustration for the managers and providers required to use these technologies. This results in reluctance or refusal to use simulation modeling and reap its benefits. Furthermore, one technological advance does not work with another. Some examples include: data collection software cannot be integrated with the database software used for building the simulation models; capacity planning solutions arrived at by using simulation software; Microsoft Visio does not meet minimum standards for health care architecture design; and simulation engineers use different software packages and the end user must learn more than one software system.

Interoperability between health care systems and simulation software is as lacking as interoperability between simulation software packages and the engineers who use them. Health care providers are not going to accept technology that changes them, is inflexible, or does not have cross-application and multidimensional input and output. If tools such as simulation modeling are to find their place as the evidence-based phenomenon they can be, standards must be set for health care providers to embrace the simulation modeling process, the tool, and the engineers who build the models. We recognize and applaud the architects, health care providers, and simulation engineers who have made efforts to use simulation modeling to improve patient care. Projects like the aforereferenced nursing time and motion study (Hendrich et al. 2008) have used a multidimensional team, with simulation modeling, to demonstrate and facilitate analysis of a robust data set. The time has come for the movement to surge forward.

Finally, the nursing perspective and role in any health care simulation modeling project is critical to its success.

References

Aiken, L.H., Clarke, S.P., and Sloane, D.M. 2002a. Hospital staffing, organization, and quality of care: Cross-national findings. *International Journal of Quality Health Care* 14: 5–13.

Aiken, L.H., Clarke, S.P., Sloane, D.M., Sochalski, J., and Silber, J.H. 2002b. Hospital nurse staffing and patient mortality, nurse burnout, and job dissatisfaction. *JAMA* 288:1987–1993.

Aiken, L.H., Sloane, D.M., and Sochalski, J. 1998. Hospital organization and outcomes. *Quality Health Care* 7: 222–226.

Aiken, L.H., Smith, H.L., and Lake, E.T. 1994. Lower Medicare mortality among a set of hospitals known for good nursing care. *Medical Care* 32: 771–787.

Anderson, S. 2007. *Deadly Consequences: The Hidden Impact of America's Nursing Shortage*. National Foundation for American Policy, www.nfap.com.

Begun, J.W., Zimmerman, B., and Dooley, K. 2003. Health care organizations as complex adaptive systems. In *Advances in Health Care Organization Theory*, eds. S.M. Mick and M. Wyttenbach, 253–288. San Francisco: Jossey-Bass.

Hendrich, C., Skierczynski, B.A., and Lu, Z. 2008. A 36-hospital time and motion study: How do medical-surgical nurses spend their time? *The Permanente Journal* 12(3): 25–34.

Heyman, P., and Wolfe, S. April 2000. *Neuman Systems Model*, University of Florida, http://www.patheyman.com/essays/neuman/index.htm.

Holden, L.M. 2005. Complex adaptive systems: Concept analysis. *Journal of Advanced Nursing* 52(6): 651–657.

Institute of Medicine. 2000. *To Err Is Human: Building a Safer Health System*. Washington, DC: National Academies Press.

Laskowski, M., and Mukhi, S. 2009. Agent-based simulation of emergency departments with patient diversion. In *Electronic Healthcare: Proceedings of the First International Conference, eHealth 2008, London, UK, September 2008, Revised Selected Papers* edited by D. Weerasinghe. 25–37. Berlin, Germany: Springer.

Law, A. 2006. *Simulation Modeling and Analysis* (4th ed.). Boston: McGraw-Hill.

North, M., and Macal, C. 2007. *Managing Business Complexity: Discovering Strategic Solutions with Agent-Based Modeling and Simulation*. Oxford: Oxford University Press.

Paley, J. 2007. Complex adaptive systems and nursing. *Nursing Inquiry* 14(3): 233–242.

Poynton, M., Beil, H., BeLue, R., Habibullah, S., Mazzotta, B., and V. Shah. August 2007. Computer terminal placement and workflow in an emergency department: An agent-based model. *Proceedings of the Complex Systems Summer School*. Santa Fe, NM: Santa Fe Institute.

Reid, P., Compton, D., Grossman, J., and Fanjiang G. 2005. *Building a Better Delivery System: A New Engineering/Health Care Partnership*. Washington, DC: National Academies Press.

Smith, M., and Feied, C. 1999. *The emergency department as a complex system*. Draft.

United States Census Bureau. 2000. *Motherhood: The Fertility of American Women, 1900-2000*. http://www.census.gov/population/pop-profile/2000/chap04.pdf.

Appendix

Following is a list of influential nursing theories and philosophies. The interested reader can find a discussion of these theories on the author's Web page for the book.

- Faye Glenn Abdellah—practice model of nursing for health for all
- Patricia Benner—humanistic model
- Anne Boykin and Savina Schoenhofer—nursing as caring
- Juliette Corbin and Anselm Strauss—trajectory model
- Bonnie Weaver Duldt-Battey—humanistic nursing communication theory
- Helen Erickson, Evelyn Tomlin, and Mary Ann Swain—modeling and role-modeling theory
- Joyce Fitzpatrick—four content concepts of person, health, wellness–illness, and metaparadigm
- Lydia Eloise Hall—core, care, and cure circles
- Virginia Avernal Henderson—assisting individuals to gain independence in relation to the performance of activities contributing to health or its recovery
- Gladys Husted and James Husted—symphonological bioethical theory
- Dorothy Johnson—behavioral system model
- Kalofissudis Ioannis—complexity nursing theory
- Imogene King—open systems theory
- Myra Estrin Levine—conservation model
- Afaf Meleis—transitions theory
- Betty Neuman—systems theory
- Margaret A. Newman—health as expanding consciousness
- Florence Nightingale—environmental adaptation model
- Dorothea E. Orem—self-care deficit theory (SCDNT)
- Rosemarie R. Parse—theory of human becoming
- Josephine Paterson and Loretta Zderad—humanistic nursing theory
- Joan Riehl-Sisca—self-concept construct
- Martha Elizabeth Rogers—science of unitary human beings
- Nancy Roper, Winifred W. Logan, and Alison J. Tierney—theory of nursing

- Callista Roy—adaptation theory
- Joyce Travelbee—human to human relationship model
- Jean Watson—theory of caring
- Ernestine Wiedenbach—prescriptive theory, a situation producing theory

Acknowledgments

I would like to thank Henry Bell (formerly of Smoky Mountain Simulation Services) for his work on the models and this chapter. He, along with Robin Clark of The Qualitative Model and Training Group, provided insight, support, and engineering oversight. Further, I would like to thank Jim Walsh of Sparta, Inc. for his teams' effort to bring Bayesian networks and agent based modeling to our clinical and architectural work, and Sara Aiello, formerly of Mark Sullivan Architects, for her work on the floor plans, distance matrices, and travel paths. I appreciate the nursing critique of Lynn D'Esmond as well as editorial assistance provided by Joshua Kilbridge. Finally, I extend a very special thanks to Eva and Erik Andersen, and my parents, Helen and Paul O'Hara who did everything else to keep me moving forward on this chapter and to the book editors, Jay Shriver, and David Eitel and project editor Jay Margolis for the opportunity and their patience and perseverance

Dedication

To Mark Sullivan (1950-2009)

This chapter and the work I have done would never have been possible without the knowledge, enthusiasm, and support of Mark Sullivan, principal and founder of Mark Sullivan Architects. Mark died quite suddenly before he could be properly cited as the champion he was for furthering the integration of architecture as a critical patient care variable. When I began working for him in 1993, he had a vision that together we could improve the way patient care spaces were designed, not only for the patients, but for the nurses and other staff working in those spaces. That vision continued through collaboration with O'Hara HealthCare Consultants, LLC.

Mark always pushed to make sure architecture was represented in an evidenced-based and regulatory manner in our simulation models. He helped us shift paradigms with his work on space commissioning and his futuristic thinking and planning on how to combine the architectural software with modeling software. He was my colleague, friend, and husband. The chapter would not have been written without him. I hope I have represented his work in the best possible way.

Chapter 7

The Physiology of Service Capacity

Pierce Story and David Eitel

Physiology: The biological science of life processes, activities and functions; the vital processes of an organism.

—The American Heritage Dictionary

Capacity, in a service system, is the ability to service demand. The structure, form, and functionality of a service system, or the physiology of service capacity, are thus the attributes the service system needs to embody to effectively meet (i.e., service) demand. However, to ascertain the structure, form, and functionality of any service system, one must first accurately ascertain the demand for which capacity needs to be available, and only then create service systems that most effectively match that demand. For dynamic, highly variable demand, we must create a dynamic and variable service capacity capable of flexing to meet the incoming demand as the demand morphs and changes. This requires an in-depth, granular understanding of the demand patterns and their downstream impacts on the demand for specific resources, such as beds and staff in hospitals, as well as the interdependencies and relationships of resources within the system. With this understanding of the demand–capacity dynamic, we can more proactively and efficiently manage the resources within the service system to match the incoming demands. This chapter reveals the thinking and necessary steps and tools required to effectively analyze, predict, and proactively manage capacity to meet dynamic demand within highly variable, complex environments such as emergency departments (EDs) and inpatient bed flow.

Introduction

Hospitals are dynamic systems and must be analyzed and managed as such. This dynamism[1] includes the interdependencies of multiple complex subsystems; the high degree of complex human interactions; process and performance variability; and the variability in community demands for resources and services. This latter *dynamic demand* is an important factor in effective management, since it ultimately drives the need for resources, processes, and operations (aka *capacity*) within our systems. As community demand for the services we offer increases, decreases, or changes, so too must the capacity we make available if we are to be efficient, cost effective, and customer focused. Importantly, this needs to occur proactively and predictively, by hour, day, week, and season, as demand dynamically shifts over hours, days, and months, such that we can more comfortably and easily manage to the variability. The more precisely we can manage to the dynamic demand, the more efficient and effective our systems become. Thus, the capability to readily and proactively flex to the variable external demand patterns, at both the hospital-wide and departmental levels, is a key component of effective capacity management, dynamic resource allocation, and optimal cost control. We must manage to service demand; and we must dynamically manage capacity.

It is important to realize that there is a significant difference between randomness/chaos and dynamism. We often view the hospital systems in which we work as dominated by randomness and chaos in which there is little that can be predicted, let alone proactively managed. In particular, patient arrivals, differing acuities and disease patterns, and so forth seem and are assumed to be random and chaotic.[2] If any patterns of demand exist in the minds of managers and staff, they are often generalized and based on a gut feeling or experience from previous periods (e.g., Mondays in the ED are always worse than Thursdays), but may not have been reliably quantified and may even be incorrect. To exacerbate the problem, the complexity driven by the interdependencies and variability of the system's internal operations amplify the variation in communal demand, making it even more perplexing and more difficult to proactively manage.

This communal variation is neither imagined nor exaggerated. The variation that creates this sensation is endemic throughout hospitals and care delivery processes. Patients simply do not become ill on a schedule, nor do surgical cases end at the top and bottom of each hour, nor does one physical exam take exactly the same amount of time as the next.

And although there is indeed variation in many of our internal processes and service systems in response to the external demand dynamics, it is often neither intentional nor optimal. Rather, *process variation* is either a belated reaction to dynamism within and outside the system, which is neither effectively anticipated nor controlled; or due to intrastaff process variation, commonly a product of inconsistencies in training, performance, and expectations, thus largely unrelated to improving performance. Therefore some of the internal process variations we experience are not strategic, planned, nor valuable.

Thus the sensation of chaos created by all types of variability, internal and external, in such a highly human and dynamic work environment is understandable. The solution to this lies in first understanding variability in the context of the communal demand. When this is achieved, an ED or hospital manager can go a long way toward providing more effective service to the communities we serve while also reducing unnecessary costs, maximizing existing capacity, and creating more caring work systems. We must therefore approach management of service capacity through a proactive understanding of communal demand.

Variability and Capacity

To better understand this variability, we should first classify it. Grouped into two of their largest attribution categories, the types of variability with which we most commonly deal are *process variation* and *demand variation*. One is relatively controllable and manageable; the latter is, for the most part, only manageable at best.[3] The sources for these two variation types are obviously different (one largely internal, one largely external and communal). This grouping allows us to understand the relative impact of each type of variation on the system at large, and how, where, and to what extent we must react. Variation that can be controlled should be, since it is logically in the best interest of work systems, efficiency, and productivity. This dictum would apply to process variation, whether in terms of process times, performance, outcomes, or consistency. Variation that cannot be controlled must at least be understood and, to the extent possible, proactively managed. It is this latter form of variation (that which can only be understood but only partially controlled, if at all) that is the subject of much of this chapter, since it is this demand variability that becomes so perplexing in the context of managing our systems and controlling our own variable internal operations. Furthermore, it is this demand variation that drives the need for variation (dynamism) in our operations, processes, and service capacity, such that we can better serve our communities. Thus, the demand variation determines the physiology of the service system. Without at least an understanding of this demand variation, the systems we design and manage, which are themselves variable, become more difficult to effectively operate. Thus, we must understand and manage to the communal demand variability to effectively optimize process variability, which will in turn help us manage that communal demand. In other words, because the communal demand is, in large part, uncontrollable, we must understand and proactively manage to that demand if we are to effectively work with and within our variable internal systems, and fully optimize the functionality of the hospital as a system.

The simple reason we worry about variability at all is capacity to serve. There is, in any system, a limit to service capacity. Service capacity is obviously a significant component of the physiology of the service system. In health care, capacity can have a number of meanings, from the capacity of a given physical space to house materials, to the capacity of an ICU to house patients at any given point, to the absolute maximum number of patients that can be processed through an ED or registration within a given time. Service capacity is inevitably limited, either by physical space, resources, time, or materials. However, demand is not as limited.[4] Furthermore, since demand is variable, the capacity required to meet and serve demand is also inherently variable, even though the actual total capacity might remain fixed. For example, the maximum number of patients passing through a registration process in a given hour may be relatively fixed (given certain assumptions and constraints), regardless of the volume of patients needing to register during that hour. If demand flexes, so should capacity, such that resources are not inappropriately allocated, wait times do not accumulate, and optimal care continues to be offered. Service capacity (capacity to serve, over some period of time), therefore, can and should flex to the demand for that service, and thus the physiology of the system should reflect that capability. In health care this can happen through resource allocation, opening and closing of space (e.g., beds), or, in the long term, the construction or shuttering of facilities. Of course, this is the case only if we want to truly optimize resource allocations (read: costs), patient satisfaction (the right care at the right time in the right place), and total system throughput (maximum flow under optimal conditions). Doing so will yield tremendous benefits, if only for the lessening of day-to-day work stress, better allocation of resources, reduced cost, and a better chance to optimize patient care. Heretofore our systems' capacity has been accepted as suboptimal, due to a number of reasons that are now being debunked by experience, for example, the "patients aren't widgets" mentality. Systems thinking now tells us concepts like efficiency of patient flow, *capacity management*, and *dynamic resource allocations* are critical to survival, good for patient satisfaction, and, fortunately, achievable.

The ability for a given system to expand and contract its service capacity will aid the system in handling the demand more efficiently and optimally, up to the point at which service capacity is fully exceeded. Even then, the variability in demand might only max out the system for a short period, such that capacity is only exceeded on a limited basis. This is the case in many health care facilities, in which an ED or post anesthesia care unit (PACU) is temporarily backed up or nurses are temporarily overburdened with work. Likewise, periods in which there is excess capacity causes inherent inefficiency due to idle workers, unnecessary costs, higher inventories, and so forth. Thus, it can likely be stated without great debate that a system that flexes its capacity just enough to meet demand at any given moment is inherently more efficient and effective than one whose capacity remains fixed. Furthermore, the capacity to service demand is, at a high level, the most expensive component of health care, since it encompasses the resources, the physical plant, and processes required to meet and serve demand. And, as is widely known, resources (e.g., staff and physicians) make up the largest cost component of operations and the physical plant the largest portion of capital expenditures. Thus, any understanding of the demand coming into the system that could help in the management of capacity, and therefore the efficiency of the operation, should be welcomed. In short, for any given system with a variable demand, capacity should vary to the extent possible or to the point that total maximum capacity is exceeded. Thus, control of a complex service system such as a hospital requires dynamic management systems capable of flexing and morphing to the internal and external environment, as it is shaped by variable community demand patterns as they change, grow, or shrink.

Patterns

But how does one manage something as variable as community demand, inherently highly variable from day to day and week to week? After all, if it were as easy as a factory producing widgets, we wouldn't have issues with health care demand or capacity, right?

Fortunately, patterns exist. In fact, patterns exist for just about everything, including chaos.[5] In health care, the patterns we must analyze are far easier to discern than those in many other complex systems, such as weather, cloud formations, magnetic fields of celestial bodies, and growth of biological systems. The patterns we seek (for example, patterns of arrivals, patterns of seasonality of illnesses, patterns of workload, and so forth) exist in the world of health care. Yes, there are variations within those patterns, and the variation can indeed be quite large. Yet, there are patterns, and within those patterns there exists significant predictability. Thus, even though the world in which we work is quite dynamic, it is not all truly chaotic. If community demand is not completely chaotic, it can therefore be understood within the context of its variation, and then, to some significant degree, predicted and managed to. Control of a complex service system such as a hospital begins with understanding the dynamic patterns of community demand. Capacity matching then has to do with the analysis of demand, and the application of solutions to allow flexing and morphing to changes in demand and external to the hospital system. Capacity matching is shaped by, and within the context of, the community demand patterns as they change, grow, or shrink.

We know instinctually that patterns exist, though we may not have quantitatively evaluated them. Nurses, for example, intuitively know that some days of the week are worse than others; that certain physicians tend to be slower and less efficient that others and thus on "their days," work will be tougher; or that certain seasons of the year are more difficult. The key is to quantify these patterns so as to discern their impacts on the system. Simply knowing the trend in averages, or the average daily variation, or the average *anything* is not good enough. We need to understand trends in the context of ranges, the variation by hour and patient type, and the variation day to day and week to week. We need to improve our quantitative analysis of demand and combine that with our qualitative and experiential knowledge of the environment, so as to develop effective solutions.

Demand Patterns and Confidence Intervals

"You just never know what is going to come into the ED!" Right? Well, actually no. Since patterns exist, it is possible to predict service and demand load based on analysis of current and historical data and the patterns found therein. This is because random does not mean unpredictable, and understanding variability is the key to prediction of even random events. From a textbook on the subject, *stochastic* means "randomly occurring." Although we cannot control the occurrences of random events, *we can predict the likelihood of their occurrence*, and the consequences of these events."[6] This means that even seemingly random events can be analyzed, patterned, and, to some degree, predicted if not managed. And as we have described, the ability to pattern and thereby predict demand is key to developing dynamic service capacity systems.

In Figure 7.1 the line represents the rate of incoming, by hour of the day, for a typical weekend day for a period of time for an ED in 2003. In Figure 7.2, the line represents the rate of incoming, by hour of the day, for a typical weekday for the same period of time for that ED. On the weekend patients begin to arrive in larger numbers earlier in the day and remain at that level of inflow much longer into the day.

So, while there is a great deal of variation in patient flow overall, there is a great deal of predictability in the arrival patterns by day of the week. Sundays

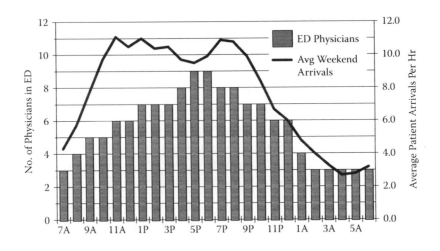

Figure 7.1 York Hospital emergency department physician staffing vs. average arrivals.

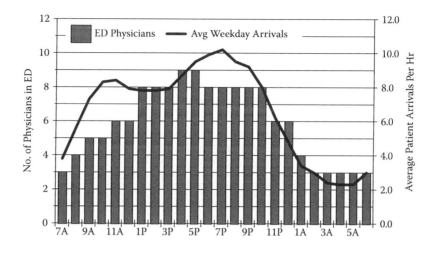

Figure 7.2   York Hospital emergency department physician staffing vs. average arrivals.

look like Sundays, and Wednesdays look like Wednesdays, within a relatively tight range of variability. Now, where do these arrival patterns (arrival distributions) come from anyway? They come from our patient registration systems. We all have them, so this kind of arrivals data is available to all of us in the ED and hospital, everywhere. But we need to also place confidence intervals around them to assist with demand analysis for capacity planning. If we merely use averages, although we will not have trouble on an average day, we will be in trouble 50% of the time when trying to meet our fairly predictable ED service loads. (Figure 7.3).

The degree and detail of the quantitative analysis that we need, and the tools necessary to use this information to effectively predict our future capacity requirements, are the next part of this chapter.

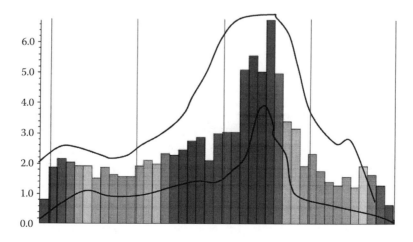

Figure 7.3   Rate of incoming with confidence intervals.

Understanding Variability: An Introduction to Queuing Theory and Simulation

Think of a restaurant, hotel, airline, dry cleaner, rental car agency, or any service business. The capacity of any given business, that is, its ability to serve customers over a particular time period, is determined by the ability to quantitatively ascertain the demand from their current and potential customer base and create the necessary capacity to meet that demand. Capacity therefore includes the resources available to the organization in the form of facilities, equipment, and labor, be it in the form of tables and cooks at a restaurant; seats on rides and food service vendors at an amusement park; chairs on a ski lift; or beds, supplies, and staff in an ED. Therefore, the demand should drive decision making regarding targets for available capacity. Otherwise, resources are wasted or opportunities to serve are lost.

We all routinely experience the results of the lack of capacity. Think of the last time you stood in line for a service (the Department of Motor Vehicles is a classic bureaucratic example). Demand exceeded available capacity and a line (or, hereinafter, a *queue*) formed. One goal of a capitalist-based and critical-to-community business is to avoid queues whenever possible. Unless you're a fan of Soviet-style economics, standing in line is not a welcomed characteristic of business transactions. Queues result in customer dissatisfaction; lost business, opportunities, and profit; increased competition (from those offering additional capacity); and the possible cost of expansion of capacity. In health care, queues might mean all of the above, with a few additional unwelcomed elements such as mortality and morbidity.

The analysis of a queue, known as queuing theory, is essentially the mathematical analysis of waiting in a line. The concepts of queuing theory have been used for decades in many industries and settings, including health care, to assess, quantify, and predict the start and "evolution" of queues over time. The goals of the study of queuing in a service system are to dissect the waits and delays in a service system and to predict, quantitatively, the service performance characteristics of the system. In particular, the system's capacity to serve under a variety of demand loads.

The core concepts of queuing are easily understood since we experience waits nearly every day in many activities (you show up, there isn't enough capacity, so you wait). The mathematics of queuing analysis, however, can be rather complicated. Complex mathematical systems and formulae have been successfully applied to a variety of settings for a variety of uses in many queuing situations. The goal of any queuing analysis is the ability to more accurately and quantitatively predict the characteristics of the systems required to successfully service demand under multiple demand scenarios.

For an ED, hospital, or other health care setting, queuing involves understanding the capacity to service the health care needs of the communities served.

Capacity takes many forms, from the number of beds in the ED, to the number of PACU spaces in surgical services, to the number of ICU (intensive care unit) beds available on a given day, or the number of parking spaces available near the outpatient clinic. All this and more must be considered for a full analysis of capacity. Analysis of queues within these systems requires us to first understand the arrival patterns of patients (the demand), and the arrival of work downstream (e.g., lab samples, radiology exams, paperwork, phone calls, etc.), so as to be predictive of all of the resources needed to manage that work. That is, the resources available to the organization in the form of facilities, equipment, and labor. The service capacity is not just about beds. In fact, it concerns all aspects of the service system simultaneously.

Analytic Queuing Models and Discrete Event Simulation

The science of queuing theory originated with a new technology called the telephone. Telephone traffic congestion was the first queuing system, studied by A.K. Erlang in Holland. In 1909 Erlang published his first work "The Theory of Probabilities and Telephone Conversations." More work on queuing theory by Erlang and others rapidly followed.

Analytic queuing models are one of the tools used in queuing analysis. They are commonly spreadsheet (e.g., Excel) or database (e.g., Access) based, and allow for some degree of variability to be studied. However, because they are inherently static and linear, their answers are inherently too limited to be as effective as is necessary when attempting to unravel the waits and delays in complex queuing (waiting) systems. On the plus side, they can be very easy to use, once constructed (i.e., put data in, get answers out). On the down side, the more dynamic one tries to make them, the more difficult they are to program, and the more difficult they become to use. Furthermore, even if some variability is constructed in the model, there are inherent constraints in their analytical capabilities, which preclude their effectiveness as analytical tools for studying large dynamic and complex systems. Although spreadsheets are useful for a number of simulation types, they simply cannot handle well queuing simulations with the existence of complexity of any magnitude. So, although queuing models can be effective in certain contexts and applications, their utility and efficacy is limited in attempts to analyze systems of any significant complexity.

Discrete event simulation (DES) modeling and DES software was designed when computers hit the scene to track discrete events as entities (e.g., patients, work, etc.) traveled through a queuing (service) system. That is, specific changes in state are tracked and time stamped as an entity moves through whatever service system is being modeled with the software. DES time clocks keep detailed track of all processing times and all waiting times, in the context of the arrival rates, which also vary over time. Through very complex mathematical analytic engines, DES models are able to explicitly represent variability, dependency, and interdependencies (= complexity) in a computer representation of any system. The modeled systems consist of entities being processed through a series of service processes and operations, with the opportunity for queues to form between each stage when there is insufficient processing capacity. This obviously is a common characteristic of EDs and hospitals.

The use of DES (and indeed queuing models) has been heretofore limited due to the resources requirements, programming intensity, and time commitments required. However, new technologies now exist that eliminate much of the difficulties associated with DES, making DES readily available as a decision support tool to users without many of its traditional constraints and difficulties.

But, why ever would an ED or hospital manager need/want a DES study to help him/her to make decisions?

The Way the World Works: A Primer on Variability, Interdependencies, and Process Simulation

Short of a battlefield, hospitals are perhaps the most dynamic, variable, and interdependent working environments. To be highly effective and efficient, all components of these dynamic systems must be in sync, but must be so within the context of variable demand, and varying patient types, staffing patterns, and workloads. In short, dynamic systems require dynamic analytical tools. Again, hospitals are dynamic systems and must be analyzed as such. Understanding and advancing change within the dynamic complexities of EDs, ORs (operating rooms), and patient flow requires dynamic and robust analytical tools. Through the effective and strategic use of DES, hospitals are now able to grasp and better manage the complex interdependencies and dramatic variability of hospital-wide patient flows. Far more analytical than spreadsheets, flowcharts, or analytic queuing models, DES gives you answers unattainable elsewhere.

Essentially, DES is the replication, in computerized form, of complex systems. Imagine, for instance, tearing the roof off an ED and looking down from above on the operations as they take place. Imagine studying all the activities, processes, and staffing from that bird's-eye vantage point. Then, imagine being able to reach down into the system and make changes to key parameters, such as staffing mix, patient volumes, processes, and so forth, on the fly, to test the impact of the changes you make as they relate to the system as a whole.

To think of it in another way, imagine being able to go to an empty field, build an exact duplicate of your OR, staff it, and use it for while. There you can change it, alter it, manipulate all the parameters in it—anything you desire to test—then study the outcomes of those changes before you take them back and implement them in your real OR.

Essentially, that is a DES simulation. Simulation is a dynamic replica of a complex working system for the purpose of thoroughly studying that system and:

■ Understanding variability and complex interdependencies via a reliable replication of the operations, systems, and changes over time
■ "Serious play" with complex possible solutions, to understand the impacts of change to the system, including the system's "next bottleneck"
■ Predictive analysis and quantification of the effects of multiple possible operational changes
■ Ongoing performance analysis and improvement
■ Studying resources, staffing, and utilization based on various scenarios
■ Deeper understanding of opportunities, system potential, and systemic bottlenecks

The power of DES comes from three main attributes, which give it the power necessary to analyze the system's functionality and conduct important what-if analyses based upon a realistic replication of the actual working system. These are:

1. The ability to account for variability
2. The ability to account for interdependencies
3. The ability to account for changes over time

These three attributes give DES the ability to reliably and accurately replicate even the most complex systems with a high degree of accuracy and legitimacy. This, in turn, allows one to conduct what-if scenarios, in which one can test options and ideas for change before they are actually implemented in the real setting.

Variability in and between Processes

Human activity is variable. That is, no two iterations of a given human activity take exactly the same amount of time. Whether it's going to the lounge to get your next cup of coffee or placing an IV in an elderly patient, there is always some degree of variability in the time it takes to complete a process or activity. Some variability is minor, some significant.[7] The degree of variability in the process or the number of times one must do the process in a given time period can have a significant impact on other activities to be completed. This is because variability inevitably reduces efficiency, total process flow, and throughput by constraining capacity over time.

Furthermore, variability within a series of processes has the effect of compounding. That is, the variability of one process directly affects the next process, and the next, and the next. This is particularly true when a process takes longer than its average process time, as it inevitably will. When this occurs, process delays occur, and the entire system becomes constrained at that point. Downstream (later) processes must wait for the previous process, now taking longer than expected, to complete. This variability can impact upstream or

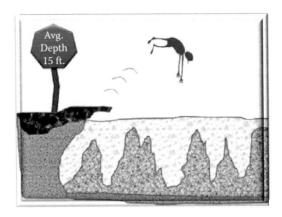

Figure 7.4   The danger of using averages.

previous processes as well by creating wait times for the next process to occur. For instance, if registration takes longer than expected, the next patient must wait; and then the next and the next. Thus variability in one process can severely alter total system process times, flow, and balance; variability impacts more than just the variable process itself—it can affect the entire system. This is commonly known as the theory of constraints[8] and can be seen in every area of our lives in which there is variability (Figure 7.4).

Essentially, variability kills throughput. Thus, it is necessary to account for relevant variability to accurately examine process parameters such as patient flow, throughput times and quantities, process times, wait times, staffing requirements, and so forth. This is particularly true in very complex environments, such as an ED or hospital. However, even our most commonly used metrics belie this important analytical need (Figure 7.4).

Analysis of systems requires metrics. These metrics are often measured and discussed as single numbers, most commonly averages. We use averages throughout health care, such as average length of stay, average daily census, and average number of arrivals (Figure 7.5).

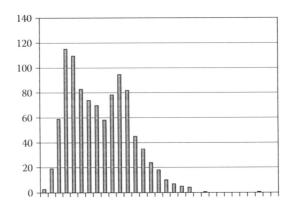

Figure 7.5   A comman type of patient arrival distribution.

However, the use of average numbers fails to account for process variability, resulting in what is called the *error of averages*, which can lead to misleading results, bad decisions, poor financial performance, and poor patient and staff experiences. Remember, patients never experience the average; they always experience the variability. As described earlier, variability alters the performance of a variable system. If the system's expectations are based on a single number, that is, the average performance of something, our estimates will inevitably be wrong to some degree (depending, of course, on the degree of variability). Thus averages tell us little about service performance, since the outliers (those activities and processes that take much longer than the average) are what "gum up" the works. Consider the long length of stay of just a few complex patients in the ED, and how those patients cause backups in other parts of the ED. Because spreadsheets calculations and flowcharts that utilize averages do not account for this important process variability, using these tools can yield misleading conclusions.

DES takes variability into account, allowing a much more realistic depiction of complex, real-life processes, and therefore more accurate predictions of throughput and other key service performance characteristics. DES uses distributions (or data curves) as inputs to represent activity and process times rather than averages in deriving results. This approach much more accurately represents activity and process times and inherent system variability. Thus, DES allows for more accuracy and realism.

Interdependencies

Because hospital processes are interrelated, changing one process affects the others in the system (Figure 7.6). Flow from the ED impacts demand for inpatient beds, constraints in discharge processing impact OR flow, radiology staffing constraints impact the EDs demand patterns, and so forth. Coupled with the

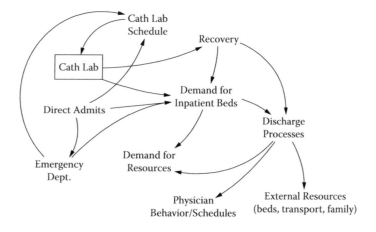

Figure 7.6 **The accurate examination of complex interdependencies is perhaps the most important element in deriving throughput and service capacity in a hospital.**

inherent, often drastic variability within processes, these interdependencies make process analysis particularly complex.

DES takes the interdependencies of processes within a system into account, thus allowing the user to see how changes to one or more processes can affect others, both upstream and downstream. Without this capability, analysis of any system-wide impacts of proposed operational changes becomes extremely difficult, particularly in complex systems such as EDs, ORs, and hospitals.

Changes over Time

Processes take place and change over time. Furthermore, external variables from patient acuities to volumes to technologies can impact processes over a day, a week, or a year, as the patterns of arrival and acuity/illness change over periods of time. For example, an ED sees a variance in patient load by hour of day, day of week, and month of year; thus, it and the rest of the hospital must react to and in anticipation of these changes over time.

To properly account for the effects of process change, particularly subtle change, one must be able to evaluate changes over a span of time. This is one of the fatal flaws of analytic queuing models and spreadsheet/database analysis. Queuing models must assume the existence of a steady state when evaluating changes to a system. DES, on the other hand, can be made to flex over time, as parameters change in the real world, better replicating the real world. Furthermore, DES models can evaluate changes over months and even years in order to determine the true long-term effects of changes to a system over long periods of time. This allows one to see how changes, combinations of change, and even subtle changes, will affect the overall system over the course of extended time periods. This is particularly helpful when analyzing new space, expanded service offerings, increased or decreased staffing allocations, and the deployment of new technologies or operational systems.

What-Ifs and Predictive Analytics

Because DES accounts for variability, complex interdependencies, and the effects of time, the models built by DES tools can be very reliable replications of even the most complex of real-life systems. With a reliable and accurate replication, we can then test various potential changes to that replication (simulation model) to determine the impacts and repercussions of changes on the system. Because of the inherent reliability and the structure of a well-constructed model, users can feel comfortable that what happens in the model will reliably happen in the real world when the changes are actually implemented.

By testing possible solutions to problems, DES becomes a risk-free environment for the evaluation of ideas and potential solutions to problems. Combinations of complex solutions can be tried in minutes using a model that might take months to implement and analyze in an ED or on a hospital floor.

Thus, DES serves as a safer, more time-efficient "predictive analysis" tool for operations management decision-making.

"Up–Down–Up" and Hospital Service Capacity

Keep in mind that when we speak of dynamic demand and capacity matching, we can be speaking at either a departmental or hospital-wide level. Heretofore, many of the efforts to fix hospital operations have been at the departmental level, such as the ED, surgical services, and radiology. Health care has adopted a number of valuable methodologies, including Lean, Six Sigma, Lean Six Sigma, CQI, and PDCA (plan–do–check–act). Their goals are all similar: fixing dysfunctional processes or systems. However, these fixes, while often helpful, might not have been made in the context of the performance of the entire system. Indeed, a repair of or alteration to the flow and available capacity in one functional area might actually have detrimental, unforeseen, and unknown impacts on another. This in turn might reduce or even negate the impacts on the functional area one tried to improve, or even negatively impact the system as a whole. For instance, improving the throughput of admitted patients from the ED might actually cause larger constraints for, say, telemetry beds during certain hours of certain days, as the OR or cath lab vie for those same resources. This is in part because many of the improvement methodologies do not deal specifically with systemic demand and capacity analysis. Indeed, some of the advocates of these methodologies have discounted the use of the very tools that can be most valuable in this systemic analysis, such as DES. Nonetheless, these methodologies will continue to be highly valuable in the grander scheme of hospital and health care service performance improvement, especially as the DES becomes more widely adopted. Health care should combine the strategies and methodologies of department-level improvement with a systemic analysis of demand and capacity, at a hospital-wide level, so as to fully evaluate and manage the entire system. Simply put, we need to be able to view our solutions as applied to the departmental level at the system level as well, so as to reliably predict the outcomes of changes to the parts as they impact the whole. Without doing so, we risk shifting demand, strains, and constraints from one functional area to another, actually worsening the allocation of resources within the system.

Demand and Capacity Matching

When we speak of demand–capacity matching and management, we need to look at the functional areas through which the demand originates (e.g., the ED or surgical services), then look at the entire hospital to analyze critical interdependencies and systemic constraints that might impair flow and impede improvement efforts. In other words, we seek the simultaneous optimization of overall hospital service performance. We need, then, an "up–down–up" approach wherein we look at systemic hospital demand and capacity, as well as the functional area/departmental demand and capacity. This will prevent us from overbuilding an ED's bed capacity without accounting for flow from the cath lab or direct admissions, and prevent the misallocation of resources (beds, money, and staff) across the spectrum of hospital services in relation to the variable demand from our communities.

The Physiology of Service Capacity

Now that we know we can analyze these complex systems in the context of their variability, we need to know how to go about it and what to do with the information. As stated earlier, the physiology of service capacity is simply the construct and function of a service system. And since demand varies, the physiology of service capacity must necessarily morph to attain a construct to enable service capacity to be maintained in the context of dynamic service loads. Whether "up" or "down," the system must dynamically change its physiology to dynamically meet the demand of the community. Therefore, what we need to construct is a physiology—a service structure and behaviors—that will accommodate communal demand.

But at what level of detail?

Granularity

As we have stated throughout, variability in the demand patterns coming from the community drives the need for dynamic capacity planning and management since the demand patterns are themselves dynamic. Thus we should analyze the demand patterns coming to/from the various areas of care (e.g., prehospital emergency services, or from the ED to an inpatient bed), accounting for the variability in the patterns, in order to construct the necessary service physiology.

In seeking to discern demand patterns, patient demand must be at the appropriate level of "granularity," or detail, as well as at the appropriate point of time. For instance, if we seek demand patterns for ED capacity, we should analyze the arrival patterns of patients coming into the ED by patient type, by hour of day, day of week, and month of year, with seasonality. If we want to analyze the demand pattern for registration, we should analyze both the scheduled and unscheduled arrivals of patients into the registration area but not necessarily by patient type. Why leave out patient type in the second example? Simply because it may not matter to this particular process. If the level of detail in the arrival pattern (in these two examples) will tell us something about the work created, resources required, length of the patient visit, process, ED operations as a whole, and so forth, then we should capture that level of granularity. If not, we can leave it out. So, since the patients' types (e.g., Emergency Severity Index (ESI) triage levels, subacuity levels such as chest pain or mental health) tell us something about the downstream resource demand caused by that arrival, we should record the patient type. However, registration processes and downstream operations might not be impacted by the type of patient being registered. Even if there is a difference in the processing time for each patient, we can account for that in a process time distribution without the hassles of accounting for each patient type. Therefore, unless the patient type itself is an identifier of current or future process variation, processing time variation, or changes in current or downstream operations, we can leave it out. If specific patient types dictate the use of additional resources for the registration process, we might want to discern the arrival patterns of those specific patient types that create additional resource demand in order to capture the variation in the demand for specific resource types.

To reiterate, we should seek the patterns in community and arrival demand that create work, demand for resources, or other critical parameters we want to study. So, for the earlier ED example, we might want to know what the arrival pattern of, say, ESI level 3 patients means for aggregate length of stay of all patients. Or, we may want to know the arrival patterns of level 3 versus level 5 patients, so as to discern the resource requirements at triage that might enable us to "treat and street" more patients from the front end. The demand must therefore be analyzed with enough specificity to answer the critical questions about the capacity, current and future, we are seeking to analyze.

In general, data should be analyzed by hour of day and day of week for each necessary grouping of patients or demand. Thus, Monday's arrival pattern for level 3 patients into the ED should be an analytical reflection of multiple prior Mondays, such that a discernable pattern might appear. ED demand should be analyzed at least hourly, and should not be aggregated into "noon census"-type data sets.

A critical component of this is the range around the mean and the confidence intervals (CIs) around the mean. This tells us the range of demand that we can expect on a given future Monday, and furthermore what demand is considered an outlier (more on outlier management later on).

Using this approach we can begin to discern the need for capacity as that need varies throughout the day and days of week. However, we must be careful to avoid seasonal variation, which might skew the data. For instance, taking a year's worth of Monday's ED arrival patterns might blend a bad winter flu season with a spike in summer orthopedics cases. If these arrivals occur for different reasons (and they well may), or if the demand patterns create different capacity requirements (and they may), or if the variability in demand is sufficient to alter the overall capacity requirements of the system we are studying, then we should break out the variation into season splits. Indeed, it is not uncommon to look at data over a month's time to try to discern intramonth variation, or variation between certain weeks.

Furthermore, extraneous circumstances such as unusual events might skew certain patterns. Variations in rural hospitals in remote areas of the Northeast can be skewed dramatically on holiday weekends, as vacationers flock to the area for short periods of time. It is thus wise to parse the data wisely and carefully, such that the patterns that arise for the analysis are valid within the context of the systemic variation and circumstances.

HODDOW WOMSOY

So, when thinking of the appropriate level of granularity, consider HODDOW (an acronym for hour of day, day of week). If weekly variation or seasonality is critical to the understanding of the variability, think additionally about WOMSOY, which stands for week of month and season of year. HODDOW WOMSOY should guide you to an appropriate level of granularity in the demand data in relation to planning for capacity requirements.

Forming a Dynamic Resource Allocation

From the demand data and an understanding of the resulting workload, we can effectively begin to build a dynamic resource allocation appropriate to the variations in demand. We do this by analyzing the demand variation with its ranges according to the level of granularity we have chosen. Assuming we have chosen that level properly, we should be able to discern the different levels of service requirements the demand is generating. Taking this to the next level, we can then begin to match resources, such as nurses with the appropriate skills or beds of a specific type, to the variable community demand.

In a simple case of the number of beds or space required, we can simply quantify the demand and its range and patterns. So, for instance, the study of spatial requirements for a mental health unit in the ED will require the simple study of the pattern of mental health patients arriving in the ED on various days and times, and the variability by hour of day, day of week, and seasonality (remember HODDOW WOMSOY).

In the case of actual human resources, this step requires a detailed understanding of the underlying processes, process times, resource utilizations, and so forth, and the downstream impacts of the demand coming in. For instance, for a given nursing unit, demand for inpatient beds creates a certain workload associated with an admission (including everything from paperwork to cleaning a room). This will likely require good process mapping and perhaps even some time–motion observation to gauge the actual work required for each demand type analyzed. So, for the admission example, a given nursing unit may want to study the processes and total time required to intake an admission (complete, of course, with variability of portions of the process and/or the entire process time). This will aid in discerning how many resources will be required to manage the given demand.

Variations in the demand and the ranges/CIs around that demand will aid in determining what is a more typical day, what constitutes predictable demand,

and what constitutes an outlier day. In the case of the bed demand example, we want to discern how many beds are demanded within, say, 80 percent of the historical, seasonal Tuesday afternoons. Or, for the inpatient bed resource analysis, we may want to analyze the variation in demand as it relates to the need for additional resources on certain days, hours, and seasons.

The outliers in the data will help us to quantitatively understand which volumes are outside an acceptable range of variability. That is, how many are outside a given pattern of range of demand. The related process, resource, and operational data can aid us in understanding the outlier demand levels that require unexpected quantities of resources (whether less or more). These may be two different numbers, however. For instance, outlier numbers of beds in demand may not exactly correlate with outlier resource demands. The range of telemetry beds within a given CI for a Tuesday afternoon between 2 p.m. and 4 p.m. may not correspond easily with the number of nursing staff required to admit patients. This might be due to the existing staffing pattern or the task allocation for specific resources, or simply that number of beds that lies outside the range (e.g., two). Thus, there may be more than one point at which the system may need to flex, based on pure numerical demand and based on the process, resource, or operational requirements of that demand. In the aforementioned case, the number of resources might be realigned based on new task allocations such that the unit can flex more consistently and uniformly, in sync with the demand for beds. Resource allocations, regardless of type, must be viewed in the context of the dynamic range of demand, the variability of internal operations, and the capacity each part of the operation is capable of offering.

Thus, from this we can begin to determine the various levels of system demand that constitute varying degrees of resource allocations, whether those be human resources (nurses and physicians) or physical resources (beds and supplies). And by analyzing the data based upon the types of downstream resource requirement the demand creates, we can focus on the level of granularity required to offer us the analytics necessary to answer our particular questions.

The Point of Appropriate Time Stamps

Before we move on from the data analysis portion of the chapter, we need to stress one more important attribute: appropriate time stamps. In order for the demand data to yield the proper analysis, we need to base it on the true demand time. *Demand time* is that specific moment in time when demand is generated or a downstream resource is required. This may be entirely different from our available information technology (IT) system's data time stamps.

Indeed, whether for value stream mapping or other analyses, many process time stamps are found to be missing as we try to locate and analyze process data. This is due to the history of health care data systems, which in large part were originally for financial analysis. Thus, in analyzing processes and operations, we often find that there are large gaps in the available data regarding operations, requiring workarounds and proxies.

This can be the case with demand time data points. For instance, what is an appropriate time stamp for the demand for a registration resource? Is it the time the patient was registered or the time of actual patient arrival? These might be two entirely different numbers, depending on the queue that awaits an arriving patient and the accuracy with which the actual arrival time is recorded. If we use the registration time, we alter the studies' demand patterns, possibly moving the demand forward in time, and smoothing it out such that boluses of arrivals are lost in hidden, unrecorded queues. As another example, what is the appropriate time stamp for an OR admission? It is not uncommon that the actual time of demand is not recorded. However, we may have a PACU arrival time, which, through additional analysis, may serve as a proxy.

Some time stamps are almost never recorded. For instance, the demand for an inpatient bed from the ED might be said to begin when the ED physician makes his or her decision to admit. However, the recorded time stamp may be the time at which the unit secretary first calls for the bed, perhaps hours later. Here, we may be able to use one of a number of proxies. One proxy might be the time stamp written or entered in the patient record stating the physician's last review of the patient chart before the admission process (which, of course, requires a tedious manual gathering process). Or, one might use the time at which the last labs and radiology reports are reviewed. Proxies are what they are—attempts to discern particular operational time stamps from related operational values. If we are fortunate, either the actual time stamp or some reliable proxy exists such that we can collect our necessary data points. Be creative with your proxies, and keep the ultimate goal of the analysis in mind as you search for substantive proxy data.

In sum, to effectively study the demand, we need to know precisely when the demand was generated, not when we begin meeting the demand with resources, or when care is initiated, or when some related processes begin. We need to discern, and gather appropriate data for, the time at which the demand in the system is actually generated either through appropriate, specific process data or some reliable proxy.

Dynamic Capacity Matching, System Balance, and Serious Play

The next three steps in the analytical process are part of what we call DCAMM™ (dynamic/demand capacity analysis, matching, and management) methodology. This methodology evolved from the use of the tools described earlier in this chapter and was born of an evolution of analytical thought that began with the use of simulation tools in typical silos and ended with the creation of hospital-wide analytical simulation toolsets. The next three steps in the DCAMM process were the logical successors to the initial demand analysis, which started as a simple simulation model.

If you have made it to this point, you should at least have a solid and better understanding of what you are facing and, at best, the demand patterns that drive the need for particular capacity requirements. Indeed, you should now have the ability to effectively study the demand for any service system, its variability, and its respective resource allocation requirements. The next step in your analysis was to evaluate the nature and specificity of those resource requirements, such that you can begin to dynamically allocate resources to match the dynamic demand.

Thus you have come to an important analytical and managerial stage, dynamic capacity matching. In this stage, the goal is predictive analysis of demand patterns, such that daily, weekly, monthly, and seasonally you can effectively predict the demand and resource requirements for as much demand as is reasonable or possible. Through the use of the analysis of the variability of demand, that is, the ranges/CIs in the demand patterns by HOWDOW WOMSOY, you should seek to discern any reasonable standardization, patterns, and consistencies that will drive future decision making on resource allocations. This ongoing analysis can reveal the patterns that will allow for more consistent scheduling of resources, a better understanding of the ranges of variability of demand for specific resources, and the overall systemic impacts of the communal demand variability. Here, too, you should begin to discern the variation between days, months, and seasons, as patterns for the various periods emerge from your analysis.

Stepping back to the dynamic resource allocation process, you can now begin to proactively and dynamically align resources, (e.g., beds, staff, and physician schedules) to match the incoming variable demand. To the extent possible, you may even try to regulate the demand for certain resources, based on systemic demands from specific sources of patients. For instance, it may be necessary to actually hold patients in the well-functioning ED during certain hours to prevent PACU backups. If this can be effectively predicted, even to within a reasonable degree of certainty, any negative impacts can be largely negated through the manipulation of capacity within specific functional areas, such as holding areas and admission units.

Before we move on with this, a note on the concept of *surgical smoothing* is worthwhile. This concept was purported by several influential authors and "gurus," and was based initially on work done at Boston Medical Center. Surgical smoothing attempts to smooth out demand variation for specific inpatient bed type by altering the surgical schedule to better accommodate inpatient bed capacity. Through smoothing, spikes for specific types of inpatient beds on "ortho day" or "cardiac day" were eliminated as cases were spread across the entire week, such that the volume on any given day was "smoother." In a sense, manipulating and limiting demand for resources is used to prevent capacity constraints.

While fine in concept, the idea commonly ran into the teeth of political buzz saws of OR scheduling, and thus was not as effective as it had been in facilities where either there was great excess capacity, or where the surgeons were more beholden to and reliant upon the hospital for OR time, such as AMCs. This meant that what might have been an effective solution for managing at least some of the systemic (and theoretically controllable) variability might not succeed as designed and intended.

More important for this topic, however, was a general failure to account for the variation, both daily and seasonally, in the demand patterns from other sources of patient demand, such as the ED or cath lab. The assumption was made that the variability was steady and consistent enough to be predicted without much effort. Therefore, it was not accounted for in the analysis of total bed demand. Without effectively accounting for the variability in demand from these areas, however, one could miss both opportunities for further improvement as well as detrimental impacts from manipulating demand in a single functional area. In other words, by failing to account for the system's total demand and variations therein, surgical smoothing did not attempt to effectively quantitatively analyze dynamic systemic demand, nor optimize total system capacity. This is a gap in the methodology for which DCAMM corrects, perhaps giving the concept of surgical smoothing a better chance of success than it might have had in some facilities where it otherwise would not have worked. Indeed, today, perhaps due to its limited effectiveness, this theory is not often discussed, and its proponents having largely moved on to other, more robust ideas.

System Balance and Critical Common Resources

As we analyze these systemic patterns of demands and the impacts on downstream resources, we come to an ability to better manage *system balance*. This means the predictive, collective analysis of those discernable and predictable demand patterns in the context of each functional area and each of their respective demand for collective resources (e.g., telemetry beds or transporters). To the extent that any demand pattern can be discerned, one should analyze them in the context of (1) the downstream resources required, (2) the functional areas immediately involved in servicing the demand, (3) the systemic demand for resources, and, now, (4) the system's "balance," as it relates to critical common resources.

For an interdependent system to effectively function, there must be balance among the components. In this case, there must be balance for demand of critical common resources across functional areas, such that the system attains and remains in balance and avoids constraints caused on the various sources of variable community demand. As was witnessed with the concepts of surgical smoothing, failure to effectively account for demand variation and patterns in all functional areas can lead to suboptimal implementation of even the most logical solutions. Thus, we must constantly analyze the entire system, looking for "variations in the variation." That is, we must constantly seek out when, where, and to what extent the patterns or the variation changes, such that the impact of such changes can be proactively managed and recorded for the sake of experiential but quantitative learning.

DES and System Balance

DES, with its ability to effectively analyze what-if scenarios, can be an effective tool in proactively managing system balance. The concept of using DES for this sort of analysis is not new to other industries, yet it is quite new to health care.

Recall that DES is capable of what-if scenarios, based on changes to the parameters of the modeled systems. For instance, one could model the impact of changes in ED volumes and acuity patterns on the resulting demand patterns for various hospital resources such as nurses or telemetry beds. Alternatively, one could study the impact of increases in mental health patient volume on constraints in ED length of stay, by day of week and hour of day. Since DES is capable of such predictive analytics, it can be quite helpful for proactive, predictive learning.

Proactive, predictive learning entails the use of predictive tools, such as models, and "serious play" around the scenarios the models are capable of creating.[9] Through the effective use of the models to play with various possible circumstances, DES can help us to understand the possible impacts resulting from changes to our key parameters. Thereby we can effectively predict, within a reasonable degree of accuracy, what might happen if certain key parameters are in some way altered.

Using these tools, then, we can proactively engage in the study of possible circumstances, using the scenarios of the DES models, such that we can understand the system reaction to parameter changes before they happen, such that if/when they actually happen, we can fashion a proper response. This is not dramatically different from the concepts of disaster planning in which live subjects pretend to be among the dead and injured in a mock disaster, so as to test the effectiveness of the response. (Of course, DES models have been quite good in these situations, when and where they have been used.) Knowing, then, the outcomes of possible circumstances, we can better respond as those circumstances arise, or better yet, even anticipate them as they begin to evolve.

From the analysis can come a better understanding of the points at which the system begins to break down, or the breaking points of the system's capacity. If we can understand the dynamics of demand, and we can ascertain the range of typical patterns from the outliers, and we can use our tools to predicatively analyze the results of changes to our systems, then we should be able to effectively analyze the points at which the parameter changes begin to result in system failure—the "breaking points" of service capacity. Armed with this information, a proactive manager can not only understand the outcomes of outlier days but see those outlier days as they begin to evolve, and act accordingly based on previous serious play and general analysis of system management and outcome control. This means a dramatic, profound, and positive change to the way many hospitals are currently managed, and will allow for the advancement of capacity enhancing changes to allow the care delivery system, as a whole, to better accommodate communal, and national, demand. We need to both manage to demand and dynamically manage service capacity.

Physiology Revisited and Summary

If we can effectively understand the demand from our communities, with its variations, by HODDOW WOMSOY, we can go to great lengths to manage the service capacity necessary to meet and accommodate that demand. By deploying the right tools, we can effectively capture and study this demand as it relates to downstream resources, such as beds, nurses, physicians, and space. By studying the relationships between demand patterns and downstream resource demand, we can begin to ascertain how, where, and to what extent capacity must dynamically flex and morph to optimally meet and accommodate the inevitable, yet predictable, demand variability. This can be done, again, by using the right tools and technologies within the context of our own internal process and operational variability, such that we respond to the variable demand appropriately and with the correct allocation of resources.

As this analysis unfolds, new opportunities emerge to enhance the management of our complex systems through predictive analysis and serious play with our dynamic, analytic models. If we can begin to predict the patterns in demand—that is, to predict 80% or more within a range of variance—we can then begin to focus on the true outlier days and manage to those, rather than managing each day as if it is an outlier. Thus we can begin to proactively keep the system in balance, as we understand how variation impacts downstream resources and capacity requirements. Through serious play with dynamic models we can predict the outcomes of changes to key parameters, such as volumes and patient types, so as to discern those critical breaking points that push the system into failure mode.

These tools and methodologies are neither difficult to understand nor impossible to implement. And while they are "tools in the tool belt" for management engineers and other performance improvement specialists, they are important new concepts that should profoundly change the way hospitals are managed— managing to demand while dynamically managing service capacity.

Notes

1. Herein, *dynamism* refers to a process or mechanism responsible for the development or motion of a system, and not the philosophic theories or systems related to forces and nature and the universe.
2. It is quite common to use a Poisson distribution to describe the arrivals into many systems, whether it is a grocery store, a bank, or a hospital ED.
3. We make the assumption here that demand should be met, whenever possible, with immediate and appropriate capacity. Demand can be "held back" through rationing of care and the limitation of service capacity, but we assume this is

neither preferable nor tolerable, particularly in the American health care system. Furthermore, by its definition, the rationing of care does nothing to actually limit or reduce demand; it merely delays it or fails to serve it.

4. Demand is limited more by the size of the community and its health than by physical or resource constraints. Demand can be altered by circumstance and changes in parameters such as demographics and overall health, but is less driven by available capacity since demand may exist, whether serviced or not, regardless of available capacity to serve it. This was the conceptual flaw in early legislative attempts to control demand via limiting capacity.

5. Chaos theory, interestingly enough, is more about patterns than about the common notion of randomness and unpredictability. For a briefing on chaos theory and the work of Lorenz et al., see http://www.imho.com/grae/chaos/chaos.html.

6. R. Bateman, R. Bowden, T. Gogg, C. Harrell, and J. Mott, *System Improvement Using Simulation*, 5th ed. (ProModel Corp., 1997).

7. Of course, one could argue that certain processes, such as entering data into a computer, or checking a patient's pulse, can take place within a relatively tight distribution of process times. This is indeed quite true. However, the aggregate human processes critical to the function of complex systems tend to be more highly variable, such as traditional ED triage, lengthy surgical procedures, and patient discharge processes, and thus should be analyzed within the context of their impact on the system's functionality.

8. The theory of constraints was introduced in the seminal book, *The Goal*, by Dr. Eliyahu Goldratt (North River Press, 1984).

9. The term *serious play* comes from a must-read book by that title, *Serious Play*, by M. Schrage (Harvard University Press, 2000). Schrage outlines, using detailed examples and logical arguments, how human creativity is enhanced through the use of prototypes. Prototypes might include a clay automobile model or a three-dimensional rendering of a new building, with which Schrage contends we can conduct serious play. In this case, we are using DES models as our venue to engage our creativity and develop solutions to respond to a variety of future circumstances.

Chapter 8

The Door-to-Doc Toolkit:
*Planning Emergency Department
Capacity for Delivering Safe Care*

Twila L. Burdick, Jeffery K. Cochran, Richard Andrews,
Mary Ellen Bucco, James R. Broyles, and Kevin T. Roche

Long waits and overcrowding in hospital emergency departments (EDs) increase patient risk. To reduce risk, a new patient flow process titled "Door-to-Doc" (D2D) was developed. D2D improves patient safety and reduces left without treatment (LWOT) rates by reducing the time patients wait to see an ED physician. To do this, D2D includes implementation of "people" and "process" tools through large-scale organizational collaboration and the use of queuing theory. This chapter describes the creation, execution, validation, and results of the D2D process and D2D Toolkit in eight diverse Banner Health EDs. Results include LWOT reduction between 35 percent and 65 percent. Last, this chapter describes the D2D Toolkit that is publically available for implementation in any ED.

Introduction

Background

Hospital EDs throughout the United States are overcrowded. A September 2004 report from the Urgent Matters Learning Network, "Bursting at the Seams," described the situation as follows: "From 1992 to 2002, the number of annual ED visits increased 23 percent in the U.S., while the number of EDs decreased by 15 percent. Many EDs are overwhelmed by the number of patients needing their services, with 62 percent of the nation's EDs reporting being 'at' or 'over' operating capacity. Almost daily, newspaper headlines across the country relay stories about patients waiting for hours in the ED before being seen and tales of ambulances being diverted from one hospital to the next due to overcrowding."[1]

Patients who leave without treatment are a symptom of overcrowded EDs and are a serious patient safety concern. LWOTs are patients who choose to leave an ED without receiving medical treatment because of long wait times and congestion. McMullan and Veser note that the average fraction of LWOT patients is typically between 3 percent and 5 percent.[2] They report that many patients who LWOT do need medical attention and are either admitted later or require emergency surgery. Rowe et al. state that 60 percent of LWOT cases "sought medical attention within one week."[3] Goldman et al. found that, of their pediatric LWOTs, 15 percent were triaged as urgent at a Canadian hospital.[4] The United States General Accounting Office's report on ED overcrowding said that at one public hospital, 46 percent of those who left before medical evaluation were judged to need immediate medical attention, and 11 percent were hospitalized within the next week.[5] Baker et al. report that 46 percent of LWOTs need immediate medical attention, 29 percent need care within 48 hours, 11 percent were hospitalized within a week, 49 percent saw a physician within a week, and some LWOTs needed emergency surgery.[6] An earlier study by Bindman et al. of public hospitals report that "at follow-up, patients who left without being seen were twice as likely as those who were seen to report that their pain or the seriousness of their problem was worse."[7] Much literature has recognized the LWOT problem have built models to predict LWOT.[2,8–11] Clearly, LWOT is a critical patient-safety concern for hospital EDs.

Problems related to overcrowded ED were increasing at Banner Health, a regional health care system based in Phoenix, Arizona. In 2003 and 2004, monthly LWOT rates were as high as 14 percent in some of its largest facilities. This issue was addressed in June 2004 by one Banner facility, Banner Mesa Medical Center, in its design and implementation of a new ED process flow called "Door-to-Doc" (D2D). Early results showed that the new process reduced the time for patients to be seen by a physician and as a result, LWOT rates decreased and safety was improved. Could this process be replicated at other facilities that were experiencing similar problems? That question provided the basis for an Agency for Healthcare Research and Quality (AHRQ) "Partnerships in Implementing Patient Safety" grant conducted by the Banner Health/Arizona State University (ASU) Partnership for ED Patient Safety.

Objectives

The overall objective of the project was to reduce the rate of ED patients leaving without treatment by implementing the D2D ED patient flow process that shortens the time patients wait to see an ED physician. The specific hypothesis was that D2D could be generalized to reduce the risk of patients leaving without treatment and thus improve patient safety at Banner Health's eight largest EDs. The process of implementing and refining D2D for the different Banner hospitals would result in a toolkit for implementing D2D in diverse EDs. The toolkit would use simple quantitative methods to adapt D2D for different patient volumes and acuities, and include tools and techniques to help staff whose work is affected by D2D make the transition.

Methods

Participants

The eight Banner Health hospitals involved in this project have EDs that vary in physical layout, staff size, patient population, acuity (injury or illness severity), and busyness. The proportion of ED patients who are treated and released to those admitted as inpatients varies with seasonal demand patterns (time of day, day of week, and month of year) within each hospital as well as from hospital to hospital. Participating hospitals were:

- Banner Baywood Medical Center, Mesa, AZ: This is a community hospital located in the far East Valley of the metro-Phoenix area with 318 licensed hospital beds, 76 of which were added in 2006. Its ED also serves Banner Heart Hospital, an 111-bed facility on the same campus. In 2006, the ED had 59,987 visits.
- Banner Desert Medical Center, Mesa, AZ: This is the largest hospital in metro-Phoenix's East Valley with 549 licensed beds. In 2006, it had 83,012 ED visits. It also houses a children's hospital.
- Banner Estrella Medical Center, Phoenix, AZ: This new facility has 172 licensed hospital beds and opened on January 14, 2005, with an electronic medical record system, including a computerized physician order entry system. In 2006, it had 65,455 ED visits.
- Banner Good Samaritan Medical Center, Phoenix, AZ: A teaching facility located in downtown Phoenix, it has 575 licensed hospital beds and 85 licensed rehabilitation/behavioral health beds. In 2006, it had 53,024 ED visits.
- Banner Mesa Medical Center, Mesa, AZ: Licensed for 258 hospital beds and 62 licensed long-term/rehabilitation/behavioral health beds, it has operated at 150 beds in recent years. In 2006, it had 34,380 ED visits.
- McKee Medical Center, Loveland, CO: This facility is located in northern Colorado and operates with 115 licensed hospital beds and 17 licensed long-term/rehabilitation beds. In 2006, it had 26,352 ED visits.
- North Colorado Medical Center, Greeley, CO: Also in northern Colorado, this is a tertiary care facility with 336 licensed hospital beds and 62 licensed long-term/rehabilitation/behavioral health beds. ED visits in 2006 were 46,750.

■ Banner Thunderbird Medical Center, Glendale, AZ: It currently has 332 licensed hospital beds and 62 licensed behavioral health beds. Its ED had 71,626 visits in 2006.

In 2003, these Banner hospitals had formed a throughput collaborative based on an approach introduced by the Institute for Healthcare Improvement (IHI). IHI defines a collaborative as "an improvement method that relies on spread and adaptation of existing knowledge to multiple settings to accomplish a common aim."[12] This existing knowledge could come from other health care organizations or from outside the industry, often in the form of "expert knowledge." Participants in IHI collaboratives are health care organizations from across the world. Because Banner Health had a number of different sites with similar capacity and patient flow issues, and some sites had made improvements that could be spread, Banner adapted the IHI improvement method to create an internal collaborative.

The Banner Health collaborative model, as described by Burdick and Cochran,[13] was designed to bring together Banner facilities to improve throughput. Annual goals related to the areas of focus for improvement were developed. Participating facilities formed local teams to analyze and address issues. Two to three face-to-face "learning sessions" were held each year during which facilities reported progress. At these sessions, expert knowledge on the "science of throughput" was presented by Jeffery Cochran, a professor of industrial engineering from ASU. His participation represented an acknowledgment that managing the capacity challenges were beyond the current level of knowledge of most health care leaders and key staff, since most were not experienced in managing under such conditions. The D2D patient flow process emerged from this collaboration. Implementing this safety innovation across several EDs was the next challenge.

The Banner Health/Arizona State University (ASU) Partnership for ED Patient Safety was formed to support the implementation of D2D. It brought together individuals with knowledge of health care operations at Banner and academics skilled in industrial engineering techniques from ASU to apply operations science to health care, including access to PhD-level knowledge that is not available inside Banner Health's internal management engineering staff. At this organization and in many others, hospital management engineers have a wide range of work, and because of this, rarely have the opportunity to focus their analytical and improvement skills on complex issues in great depth, even when they recognize the need for applying scientific-based operations methods. Cochran's interest in applying tools that had been successfully used in other industries to health care coincided with the need for health care to address the increasing complexity of operating in a capacity-constrained environment. The partnership was based on creating learning opportunities for health care staff and engineering students, making the application of engineering tools accessible to health care leaders to meet new challenges, and further developing the science of health care engineering through research.

Implementation

Implementation of the D2D process flow in participating facilities was based on a model for effective change[14] that requires the development of robust technical solutions or processes along with acceptance of the change by the people affected.

People

Acceptance of the changes in the ED patient flow was addressed by engaging a broad range of individuals at various levels of the organization who recognized the need for improvement and the possibilities for great improvement outcomes by implementing the new processes. To focus attention and avoid competing ED improvement activities, a number of ED-related activities were consolidated within the D2D implementation. This included clinical automation implementation, labor productivity improvement, clinical risk interventions related to discharge, planning for new hospitals and EDs, physician call coverage, and behavioral health patient care and placement.

Organizational structures to support the project were established when the system oversight team formed first. It included administrative leaders responsible for ED operations at each of the participating facilities, along with corporate leaders. The system chief medical officer served as the executive sponsor for this group, initiating the process by extending invitations to the appropriate participants. Two members were selected to lead the team based on their interest and influence, including a chief operations officer from one facility and an ED physician leader from a different hospital. The group met twice monthly as it organized commitment for moving forward. The group described the need for change using consistent performance data from all the facilities that showed high LWOT rates. It used the success of early adopters to articulate the improvement that was possible with D2D implementation. They were able to ensure broad organizational support by making D2D a strategic initiative that was tied to the management incentive program.

A support team facilitated the process design and implementation work. Members included internal management engineers, an ASU engineering professor and two PhD students, project managers, strategic planners, clinical automation staff, organizational development, and others. As the implementation progressed, one of the ED directors joined the team as a full-time project coordinator. The support team provided consultation regarding implementation of the new model at the facility level as well as systemwide reporting of performance.

The design team, consisting of staff members and physicians from participating EDs, completed the design work. Using the D2D process developed by Banner Mesa as a starting point, the design team further refined the process based on benchmarking with other organizations. Its charge was to define an ED patient flow process that would be used consistently across Banner EDs, supported by clinical automation, and have consistent measures of success in several dimensions, including patient safety, clinical quality, patient satisfaction, productivity, and financial results. It convened over the course of six weeks in late 2005 and reached consensus on a systemwide "franchise" model that was presented to the oversight team and other stakeholders for approval. An implementation kickoff meeting was held in January 2006 for facility ED leaders with facility implementations following over the next eighteen months.

Process

The D2D process improves ED throughput by increasing the capacity of space-limited EDs and focusing on serving patients quickly. The main feature of the new process, shown in Figure 8.1, is that patient flow is split into "less sick" and "sicker" patient subgroups based on the standardized Emergency Severity Index (ESI).[15] This has the advantage of keeping less sick patients, who are the vast majority, flowing (rather than waiting in the lobby), especially during busy times. It changes the idea that all ED patients, regardless of acuity, own a bed during their ED stay.

Key features reduce the delay in seeing a physician, which in turn reduces patient loss. Upon arrival, patients are asked a few key questions to streamline the registration process. Completion of registration information follows as the patient moves through the care process. Patients then receive a "quick look"

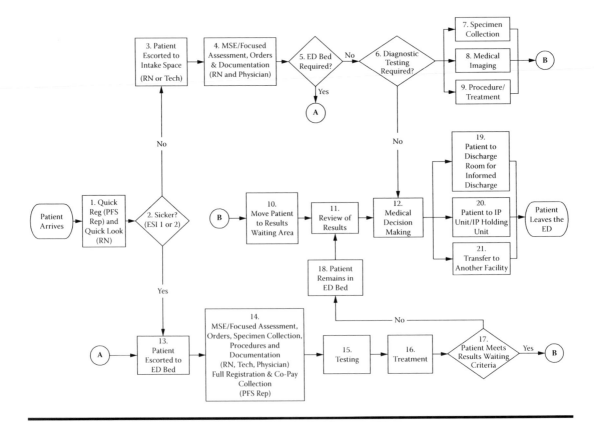

Figure 8.1   Door-to-Doc care process.

triage process, rather than the traditional extended triage. Preparation for seeing the physician is decreased as patients who are less sick may remain dressed and stay vertical rather than being placed in a bed. For those who are less sick, joint medical assessment and documentation by the nurse and physician together is encouraged. Not only does this parallel (rather than sequential) process reduce the number of steps before the patient sees the physician, it also enhances the work of the care delivery team as the members focus together on the patient, sharing the assessment process from their unique clinical perspectives.

Less sick patients do not own an ED bed; rather they move among treatment areas as they would in a clinic setting. To the degree possible, patients with lower acuities move to testing/treatment areas rather than continuously occupying an ED bed. They wait for their lab and other test results outside of the flow of other patients, in chairs or loungers, allowing better use of limited ED capacity and quicker access to physicians, returning to an ED space for discharge. The foundation for these process changes is referred to as the "bed ahead" concept, the idea of continually anticipating and creating a place with resources for the physical evaluation of the next patient.

As facilities prepared for implementation, they needed information about adapting the flow model to their unique patient acuities and volumes. ASU engineers used queuing theory, the mathematical study of waiting in lines, and queuing network analysis (QNA) as the unifying modeling approach. Based on discoveries during the modeling and data analysis that EDs are generic in a number of ways such as time pattern of arrival, relative time spent by acuity level on a patient, and the applicability of queuing, the D2D queuing model was developed. Individual facility data is entered into the model to customize the split flow D2D for different EDs. Figure 8.2 shows the D2D flow pattern when viewed from a systems engineering perspective.

In Figure 8.2, all inbound patient flow comes through Quick Look, where patients are split between Intake/Discharge (OP_{ED}) and Inpatient ED (IP_{ED}) areas based on acuity. The percentages of lower acuity patients (r_{RO}) and high acuity patients (r_{RI}) used in the model are based on facility-specific ED patient population data. Using ESI scoring, lower acuity patients are considered levels 3, 4, and 5 (shown as f_3, f_4, and f_5) and higher acuity patients are levels 1 and 2 (shown as f_1 and f_2). After seeing a doctor in Intake, a fraction of patients are determined to be sicker than was first thought and sent from Intake to the IP_{ED}. This fraction is denoted as f_{RE}; early users of split flow D2D have found up to 20 percent of patients may be so transferred. By definition, all level 3 and 4 OP_{ED} patients require tests and thus visit Results Waiting, shown as r_{OW}.

The remainder of the ED flow addresses patients who need inpatient care and those who can be discharged home. The probability that a patient will transfer from the IP_{ED} to Inpatient Transitional Care (r_{IH}) is based on the overall percent of patients admitted to the hospital from the ED (f_A), found from hospital emergency department data sources. All patients who visit the IP_{ED} that do not get placed in Inpatient Transitional Care are assumed to be discharged. Similarly, all

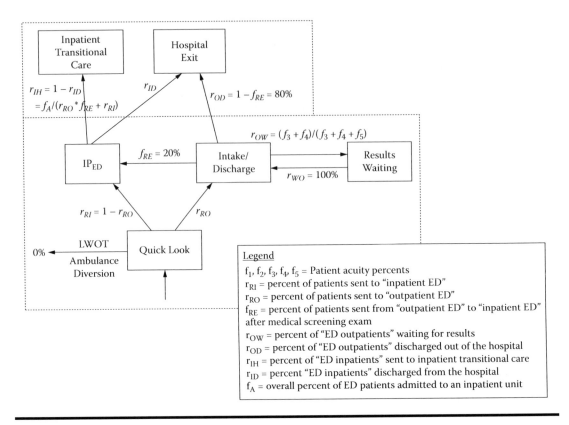

Figure 8.2   Calculating D2D flows.

patients who visit OP_{ED} who are not transferred to the IP_{ED} are assumed to be discharged. Arriving patient volumes for each facility are determined using recent experience reflected by hospital data, or future volume forecasts that represent a planning volume. These numbers must include patients who currently LWOT reflecting the goal of safeguarding patients by providing capacity for them. The division of daily volume between ED peak and off-peak hours is key to this analysis. Observations in this study and confirmed in the literature[16] show a stable 12-hour peak period from 9 a.m. to 9 p.m., including 65 percent of the day's patient arrivals. Multiplying peak and off-peak arrival rates throughout the flow network produces hourly flow arrivals to each area.

Area capacities are determined in units of physical patient space, including "entourage" space for people accompanying patients. Staffing capacities are standard ratios in the more acute side of the ED and determined by QNA for the less sick side. Historical data is used to find patient LOS (length of stay) service time distributions. Utilization targets may come from either existing industry standards or queue measures. LOS and utilization target values are input into the utilization queuing equation and solved for the required number of spaces needed to achieve the target utilization and service levels. This process is repeated for each node in Figure 8.2.

Although QNA is a highly mathematical method, in practice it is easy to use and can be implemented in a spreadsheet format wherein the mathematical formulas are transparent to the user. QNA treats each of the areas in the ED as a location where a waiting line could occur, and supports decisions about how much resource should be in each area from a "whole system" perspective. With QNA, predictions of many important performance measures are possible using key patient safety performance measures as queuing performance measures. For example, Server Utilization (ρ), which is the average percent of time a resource is "busy," includes bed utilization (the average percent of time a bed is occupied by a patient) and provider utilization (the average percent of time spent in direct patient care). Wait in Queue (Wq) is the average length of time a patient will spend waiting for service in an area before starting service. Full/Busy Probability (pc) is the fraction of arriving patients who must wait in an area until a resource becomes available. In practice, deciding upon the right performance measures for an area is a matter of trading off desired performance with capacity budget, but literature exists to provide some guidelines for utilization, wait times, and full/overflow probabilities.[17-20]

In addition to predicting the performance measures already described, D2D time can also be calculated. Table 8.1 shows sample output for one facility. In the example, estimated D2D time is just over 20 minutes during peak volumes with 2 Quick Look triage providers, 6 physicians or other licensed independent providers serving 18 intake rooms, having 30 spaces for results waiting, 20 inpatient ED beds, and 10

Table 8.1   D2D Service Level Summary

Area	Volume/ Hr	Average LOU (min)	Number of Servers	Utilization	Waiting Time (min)	Full/Busy Probability
Quick Look			1 server	>100%		
Quick Look	12.62	7.5	**2 servers**	78.9%	6.40	32.6%
Quick Look			3 servers	52.6%	0.73	14.6%
Intake/Discharge			5 docs, 15 rooms	86.9%	6.53	23.0%
Intake/Discharge	23.08	11.3	**6 docs, 18 rooms**	87.4%	1.42	14.3%
Intake/Discharge			7 docs, 21 rooms	62.1%	0.44	8.1%
Results Waiting			29 spaces	77.7%	2.55	3.4%
Results Waiting	11.27	120.0	**30 spaces**	75.1%	1.51	2.5%
Results Waiting			31 spaces	72.7%	0.89	1.8%
IP$_{ED}$			19 beds	74.0%	3.25	4.9%
IP$_{ED}$	3.36	238.0	**20 beds**	70.1%	1.67	3.3%
IP$_{ED}$			21 beds	66.6%	0.84	2.2%
Inpatient Transitional Care			9 beds	67.4%	16.44	7.8%
Inpatient Transitional Care	2.78	131.0	**10 beds**	60.7%	6.39	4.5%
Inpatient Transitional Care			11 beds	55.2%	2.50	2.4%

inpatient transitional care beds. A 5-minute transportation time is assumed for moving patients from Quick Look to the Intake area and from Quick Look to the IP_{ED}. The queuing-based formulation for the split flow network has been documented in the literature.[21] Additionally, more in-depth queuing network formulation and analyses have been performed in generalized split flow emergency departments.[17,22,23]

Measurement

Standardized measurement with consistent data elements was developed to monitor results. An ED scorecard with side-by-side comparisons of facility performance in dimensions of patient safety, quality, patient satisfaction, process efficiency measures, labor productivity, and financial results was produced monthly. The scorecard provided information for the system ED oversight team and facility ED leadership team to monitor their performance over time in comparison with other facilities. In addition, a tool for monitoring the consistency of the model after implementation across the facilities was developed. It is referred to as a *gap analysis*. This tool provides a basis for accountability as well as making ongoing improvements in the new D2D model.

Results and Interpretation

The D2D model has been implemented at eight large Banner EDs, and LWOT rates have declined at all facilities. Figure 8.3 compares performance pre- and postimplementation rates. It shows that the facility that implemented D2D with an already low LWOT rate was able to reduce these rates by 35 percent and those with higher LWOT rates saw improvements of up to 65 percent. By February 2007, the first five facilities to implement D2D had provided care for more than 12,000 patients annually who would have left without treatment prior to the implementation of D2D.

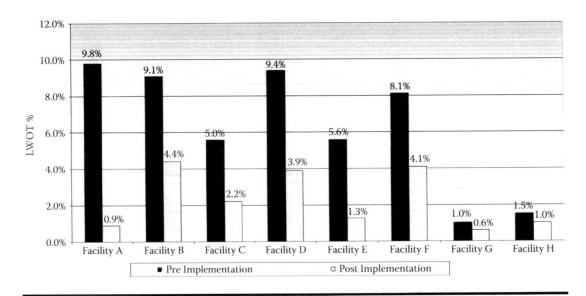

Figure 8.3   Pre/post Door-to-Doc implementation LWOT rates.

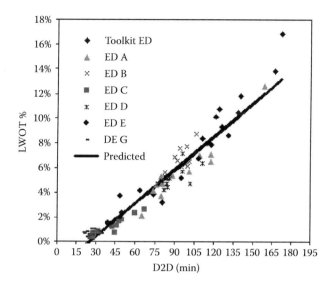

Figure 8.4   High correlation between D2D and LWOT percent.

The D2D model has decreased the D2D durations and, as a result, decreased LWOT. The D2D duration is the time between patient arrival and seeing a physician. A linear regression model between the D2D durations and LWOT percent explains 93 percent of the data (0.96 correlation coefficient; Figure 8.4). This indicates that the reduction in D2D durations decreased LWOT and increased patient safety.

An unintended consequence of the D2D process was an initial increase in patients leaving against medical advice (AMA) was observed that countered the decrease in LWOT rate. The AMA patients are the patients who have already seen a physician, received some treatment, and have left before the physician disposition. In most facilities the AMA rate returned to the preimplementation rate after a short time leading us to believe it was caused by the learning curve. In the facilities that did not staff according to the D2D model recommendation, AMA rates have remained two to four times higher than facilities that staff to the model.

After implementation of the D2D model, Banner saw an 11-percent ED LOS decrease across its system of hospitals. This reduction was purely a result of a decrease in D2D time. One of the unaddressed challenges of the D2D process was the managing of patients who were treated in the Intake Area while they were waiting for results or receiving treatment. This provides an opportunity of standardizing test and treatment processes to further reduce LOS.

Because of more rapid assessment, there were more patients being treated per physician. Traditionally, ED physicians' workload was six to eight patients concurrently. With D2D, the ED physicians can treat ten to twelve. As a result, they needed help in prioritizing patient assessment and discharge using a "zoomer" nurse. The zoomer nurse ensures that the physician has the correct patient in the correct location at the correct time. The role of the zoomer will help to facilitate flow in the Intake Side of the ED.

Discussion

Implementation of D2D began in late 2005 after reaching consensus on the design, and at each facility, both people and process implementation issues have been addressed. The timing of implementation took into account facility change readiness factors such as the urgency of ED issues as well as leadership at the department and administrative levels. Some facilities with interim or unstable ED leadership delayed implementation while they took steps to stabilize leadership first. Obtaining the appropriate levels of physician staffing caused delays or limited time of day implementation in some facilities.

The D2D model has started a paradigm shift both in process and approach to throughput improvement in the ED. Clinical providers have always used data in medical decision making but have not used data to drive operational change. Queuing theory is new to many hospital systems especially to nonteaching hospital systems. As a result, clinicians were reluctant to initially accept and use the queuing modeling to change the ED process. Through Banner Health's persistence, demonstration by early adopters, the ED redesign system initiative, and process improvement accountability (physicians, directors, etc.), this reluctance was overcome. Even facilities that had low LWOT rates prior to D2D implementation recognized that, in addition to improving safety, D2D could be useful in preparing them for the opening of a competitor facility in the community or meeting the challenge of volume growth (anticipated and surge).

On the process side, the D2D queuing model with facility-specific data was made available to guide implementation planning. Space constraints at some facilities impacted the model's full implementation, but remodeling plans have been developed to optimize D2D. Using the facility data and the model, some EDs decided to split patient flows four ways: sicker adults, less sick adults, sicker pediatrics, and less sick pediatrics. In most cases, facilities were surprised by the percentage of patients that could be seen in the Intake areas.

A continuing evaluation of D2D at Banner facilities indicates that there are additional opportunities for improving ED patient care. As previously mentioned in the "Results and Interpretation" section, overall length of stay can still be reduced by working to streamlining the results waiting process. In some facilities, staffing needs to be better matched to peak volume hours. Transitional inpatient care is a continuing challenge.

D2D Toolkit

The generic nature of EDs allowed the translation of the Banner implementation experience into a D2D Toolkit[24] for broader use. Figure 8.5 is an overview of the D2D implementation process and the tools that are available.

With these tools, users can add their facility data to a spreadsheet to learn whether they have an LWOT problem. If they determine that they do, they may

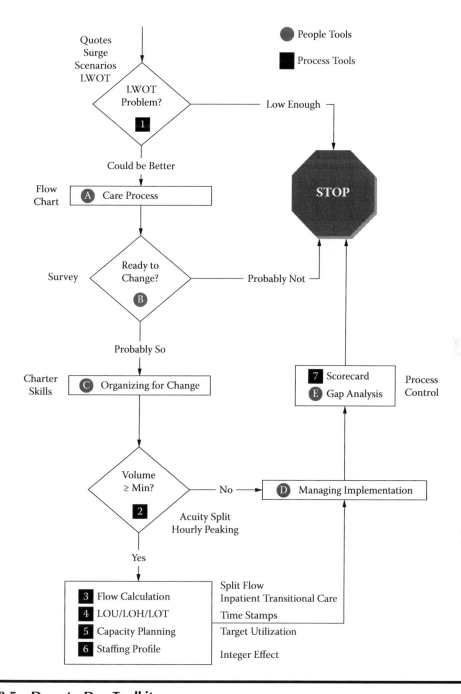

Figure 8.5   Door-to-Doc Toolkit.

want to consider adopting D2D so there are tools for comparing their current ED care process to the D2D patient flow. Based on this information, a facility will assess whether it is ready to make the kinds of changes necessary for successful implementation using a change barometer. If the decision is made to proceed, the next tool is designed to assist the facility with organizing for change. Then comes an interactive tool to determine whether volume is sufficient for splitting the patient flow. If it is, a series of spreadsheet-based tools are included to calculate arrival rates, and summarize length of use, length of hold, and length of test turnaround that are important for the next step, which is capacity planning. After capacity decisions are made, appropriate staffing is calculated in the next tool. Finally, a facility is ready to implement, and project management tools are included to assist with this step, which is followed by ongoing process and outcome measurement.

Another important implication of the success of this project is the development and use of a partnership between hospital organizations and university-level engineering resources that demonstrates the potential for such collaboration. Although this intervention and its associated tools work for any ED, its applicability may be limited by access to current ED data, which is difficult to obtain without a computerized data system and defined data extracts. Industrial engineers or others who are trained in the theory and use of queuing and other operations research techniques are also important resources.

Conclusions

D2D improves patient safety in EDs by having patients seen by a doctor sooner, thus reducing the rate of patients who leave without treatment. This was accomplished by redesigning ED patient flow using input from ED staff and physicians as well as industrial engineering methods and tools, most notably applying queuing theory. This application, developed by an ASU system engineering professor and his students, contributed to a more robust design and most appropriate adaptation of the design to local patient volumes and acuities. The technical design was complemented by strategies for acceptance of the new design that included broad involvement of frontline staff and physicians as well as leadership and other stakeholders that have led to implementation of the new D2D split patient flow model. Ongoing monitoring of the implementation and a balanced set of outcome measures continues and contributes to ongoing improvement of the design.

The D2D Toolkit translates the Banner experience into tools for implementation at other facilities. These tools allow EDs to predict patient flow rates, which is useful in allocating resources such as beds, waiting spaces, and staff to each area. The models allow ED leaders to consider target utilization for ED resources and how those decisions affect service levels and ultimately patient safety as one of the consequences of patient waiting.

Acknowledgments

This project was funded under grant number HS15921-01 from the Agency for Healthcare Research and Quality, U.S. Department of Health and Human Services.

References

1. Wilson MJ, and Nguyen K. Bursting at the Seams: Improving Patient Flow to Help America's Emergency Departments. Urgent Matters: The George Washington University Medical Center School of Public Health and Health Services Department of Health Policy, September 2004.

2. McMullen JT, and Veser FH. Emergency department volume and acuity as factors in patients leaving without treatment. *South Med J* 97(8):729–733, 2004.

3. Rowe BH, Channan P, Bullard M, Blitz S, Saunders D, Rosychuk RJ, Lari H, Craig WR, and Holroyd BR. Characteristics of patients who leave emergency departments without being seen. *Acad Emerg Med* 13(8):848–852, 2006.

4. Goldman RD, Macpherson A, Schuh S, Mulligan C, and Pirie J. Patients who leave the pediatric emergency department without being seen: A case-control study. *CMAJ* 172(1):39–43, 2005.

5. United States General Accounting Office. Hospital Emergency Departments: Crowded conditions vary among hospitals and communities. Report to the Ranking Minority Member, Committee on Finance, U.S. Senate, March 2003.

6. Baker DW, Stevens CD, and Brook RH. Patients who leave a public hospital emergency department without being seen by a physician: Causes and consequences. *JAMA* 266(8):1085–1090, 1991.

7. Bindman AB, Grumback K, Keane D, Rauch L, and Luce JM. Consequences of queuing care at a public hospital emergency department. *JAMA* 266(8):1091–1096, 1991.

8. Broyles JR, and Cochran JK. Estimating Business Loss to a Hospital Emergency Department from Patient Reneging by Queuing-Based Regression. IIE Industrial Engineering Research Conference, CD-ROM, Memphis, TN, 2007.

9. Green LV, Soares J, Giglio JF, and Green RA. Using queuing theory to increase the effectiveness of emergency department provider staffing. *Acad Emerg Med* 13:61–68, 2006.

10. Broyles JR. Industrial Engineering in Hospitals: Framework, Practical Experience, and Resources. Honors college thesis, Arizona State University, May 2005.

11. Polevoi SK, Quinn JV, and Kramer NR. Factors associated with patients who leave without being seen. *Acad Emerg Med* 12:232–236, 2005.

12. Institute for Healthcare Improvement. The Breakthrough Series: IHI's Collaborative Model for Achieving Breakthrough Improvement, Institute of Healthcare Improvement White Paper, 2003.

13. Burdick T, and Cochran JK. Collaborating to Address Capacity Constraints. Proceedings of HIMSS Annual Conference, San Diego, CA, February 13–16, 2006.

14. Palmer B. *Making Change Work.* Milwaukee, WI: Quality Press, 2004.

15. Gilboy N, Tanabe P, Travers DA, and Eitel DR. *Emergency Severity Index, Version 4: Implementation Handbook* (AHRQ Publication No. 05-0046-2). Rockville, MD: U.S. Department of Health and Human Services, Agency for Healthcare Research and Quality. May 2005.

16. HealthTech Briefing Report. Key trends in emergency and trauma services. Health Technology Center, October 2006. http://www.healthtechcenter.org/

17. Cochran JK, and Roche KT. A multi-class queuing network analysis methodology for improving hospital emergency department performance. *Comput Oper Res* 36(5):1497–1512, 2009.

18. Cochran JK, and Bharti A. Stochastic bed balancing of an obstetrics hospital. *Health Care Manage Sci* 9(1):25–39, 2006.

19. Cochran JK, and Bharti A. A multi-stage stochastic methodology for whole hospital bed planning under peak loading. *Int J Indust Syst Eng* 1(1/2):8–36, 2006.
20. Cochran JK, and Roche KT. A queuing-based decision support methodology to estimate hospital inpatient bed demand. *J Oper Res Soc* 59(11):1471–1482, 2008.
21. Roche KT, and Cochran JK. Improving Patient Safety by Maximizing Fast-Track Benefits in the ED: A Queuing Network Approach. IIE Industrial Engineering Research Conference, CD-ROM, Memphis, TN, 2007.
22. Roche KT. Whole Hospital Analytical Modeling and Control. PhD dissertation, Arizona State University, August 2008.
23. Burdick TL, Cochran JK, Kisiel S, and Modena C. Banner Health/Arizona State University Partnership in Redesigning Emergency Department Care Delivery Focusing on Patient Safety. 19th Annual IIE Society for Health Systems Conference, CD-ROM, New Orleans, 2007.
24. Burdick TL, Cochran JK, et al. Door-to-Doc (D2D) Patient Safety Toolkit. Rockville, MD: Agency for Healthcare Research and Quality. http://www.bannerhealthinnovations.org/

Chapter 9

Forecasting the Demand for Emergency Department Services

Murray J. Côté, Marlene A. Smith, David Eitel, and Elif Akçali

Introduction

Emergency department (ED) medical directors and hospital administrators could benefit from the forecasting of ED service loads so as to allow for improved ED capacity planning. Forecasting can be done to support for strategic, tactical, and operational decision making. Strategic planning has to do with long-term decision making to determine the physical size and capability of a facility. Tactical planning is for intermediate-term decision making to set staffing and resource levels and determine expected budgets. Operational planning is for short-term decision making for scheduling employees and real-time adjustment to their schedule.

This chapter will introduce the interested medical director and hospital administrator to an operations management toolset called statistical forecasting. These methods could be mimicked to allow hospital leaders to forecast the demand for ED services at their institution, with some help from someone trained in statistical forecasting. The outputs from such forecasting models can then be used as inputs for capacity planning models (e.g., Akçali, Côté, and Lin, 2006) and staffing/scheduling models (Wright, Bretthauer, and Côté, 2006).

Using a case study approach, we will:

1. Describe the arrival process to an ED
2. Decompose the arrival process by appropriate time units relative to strategic, tactical, and operational decision making
3. Demonstrate the efficacy of basic forecasting models with different planning horizons

Getting a Handle on ED Arrivals

ED arrivals can be represented by a rate of arrival per time period, type call, by hour, day, week or month. Further, additional issues that may arise when examining ED arrivals include arrival behavior (i.e., likelihood of staying in the ED or leave before being seen by medical personnel), length of stay in the ED, and likelihood of hospital admission.

Case Study: York Hospital, York, Pennsylvania, Calendar Years 1997–2006

Background

York Hospital is a 466-bed (422 licensed) community teaching hospital, serving a population of 481,000 in south central Pennsylvania. There were 3,400 employees. The ED at York Hospital includes critical care, intermediate care, and urgent care areas, three dedicated trauma bays, and a behavioral health area.

Full ancillary support services are available with trained ED nurses, many with certification in emergency nursing, emergency care technicians, patient support specialists, patient representatives, and other support staff present 24 hours a day.

Classification of ED Demand by Triage Level (Using ESI v. 3)

The York Hospital ED used the Emergency Severity Index (ESI) five-level triage during the majority of the study period. Indeed, York Hospital is one of the birthplaces of ESI triage. ESI triage (Figure 9.1) conceptually approaches the classification of patients on arrival in the following manner:

Who needs to be seen first?
   Level 1—Is this patient physiologically unstable, dying?
   Level 2—Is this a patient who should not wait?

Then, how many resources is this patient *likely* to need to get to a disposition, where resources have been classified?
   Level 5—None. Only the examination by the doctor/nurse team is predicted.
   Level 4—One resource is predicted to be needed.
   Level 3—Many: two or more resources are predicted to be needed.

Interrater and test–retest reliability has been demonstrated to be very good with the use of ESI triage, when staff are well trained and retrained. Therefore we believe the triage data contained in the York ED database for the years assessed were reliable for this analysis.

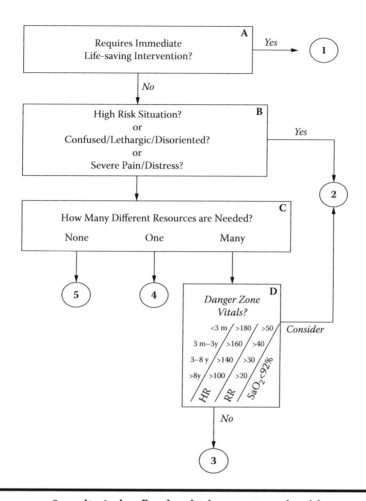

Figure 9.1 **Emergency Severity Index five-level triage system algorithm.**

We have two types of data for analysis in the database: daily and hourly arrivals to the ED. Daily data track arrivals to the ED by day and by triage level from July 21, 1991, to July 26, 2007. The daily data can be aggregated by month and year to provide intermediate and long-term forecasts. Hourly data for arrivals and by triage, covering December 1, 1999, to August 22, 2004, are used for short-term forecasting. The variable to be forecasted, named *Arrivals*, is all patients who present to the York Hospital ED and are treated and either discharged from the ED or admitted to the hospital. Off-site urgent care and express admissions were not included in the *Arrivals* variable.

The ED Arrivals Database contained the following:

- Arrivals by day and by triage from July 21, 1991, to July 26, 2007 (5,804 daily observations)
- Arrivals by hour and by triage from December 1, 1999, to August 22, 2004 (40,904 hourly observations)
- Discharge disposition (i.e., admit to hospital or discharge home)
- Sojourn (in minutes) in ED

The hospital fiscal year follows the academic calendar year, that is, July 1 through June 30.

Forecasting Using Regression Analysis

We advocate the use of regression analysis to forecast ED demand. Regression is a versatile statistical procedure capable of handling a wide variety of data patterns. Regression tools are ubiquitous and regression results are easy to understand and interpret.

The regression model that we will reference throughout this chapter includes one dependent variable, *Arrivals*, and a set of independent variables, labeled *X*. The regression model can be written as

$$Arrivals = b_0 + b_1 X_1 + b_2 X_2 + \dots b_k X_k + \varepsilon,$$

where least squares is applied to data for *Arrivals* and the *X*'s to obtain numerical estimates for b_0 through b_k. (ε is a random error term.) Once the regression estimates for b's are obtained, out-of-sample values for *X*'s are substituted into the regression equation that then generates forecasts for *Arrivals*. This general form will serve all of our forecasting needs. The numerical values for the *X*'s will be stipulated to meet the modeling needs. In all instances, though, regression is used to estimate the model and produce the forecasts.

In the regression equation, the estimate for b_0 is interpreted as the expected value for *y* when the independent variables are set to zero. The estimate for b_1 is the expected impact on *Arrivals* when X_1 changes by one of its units and similarly for the other b's. R^2 and the standard error of the regression (SE_{reg}) are two important statistics related to regression analysis. R^2 measures the percentage of variability in *Arrivals* accounted for by the model; higher R^2 values, up to a maximum of 100 percent, indicate better goodness of fit. The SE_{reg} is an estimate of the typical error in the model. Its unit of measurement is number of *Arrivals*; smaller values mean closer cohesion between the observed data and the predictions produced by the regression model. We provide illustrations of proper interpretation of these regression statistics in the examples that follow.

For producing and managing forecasts of emergency department demands, we propose a four-step procedure:

1. Visually examine the time-related patterns in the data to guide in selecting an appropriate forecasting methodology.
2. Use regression to estimate the model. Examine the regression statistics to assess the quality of the regression model.
3. Generate forecasts using regression.
4. Update the forecasts periodically as new information becomes available.

In what follows, we use the data from York Hospital's ED to illustrate this procedure.

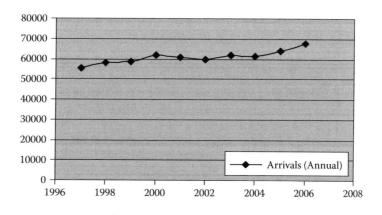

Figure 9.2 Annual visits to the York Hospital ED, 1997–2006.

Forecasting Annual Visits for Strategic Planning: Physical Capacity Needs

For the purposes of long-term planning, we calculated total number of arrivals for each of the years 1997 to 2006. We wish to generate forecasts of annual visits for 2007 to 2009. The average number of annual visits from 1997 to 2006 is 60,947 visits per year.

The first step involves examining the relevant data for time-related patterns. The *time plot* is shown in Figure 9.2, in which the data display a mostly linear, upward-trending pattern. To model linear trends, a *trend-line regression* model is appropriate; the independent variable contains the years covered by the historical period. In our case, *Year* is 1997, 1998, ..., 2006:

$$Arrivals\ (Annual) = b_0 + b_1\ Year + \varepsilon.$$

The estimated regression model is shown in Table 9.1 The R^2 of 80.0 percent means that 80 percent of the variability in annual visits is accounted for by the

Table 9.1 Regression Results of Annual Visits

Predictor	Coef	SE Coef	T	P
Constant	−1942688	354564	−5.48	0.001
Year	1001.1	177.1	5.65	0.000
New Obs	*Fit*	*SE Fit*	*95% CI*	*95% PI*
1	66453	1099	(63918, 68988)	(61959, 70947)
2	67454	1259	(64551, 70357)	(62743, 72165)X
3	68455	1423	(65174, 71736)	(63502, 73408)X

Note: The regression equation is: Arrivals (Annual) = −1942688 + 1001 Year. S = 1609.03; R-Sq = 80.0%; R-Sq (adj) = 77.5%.

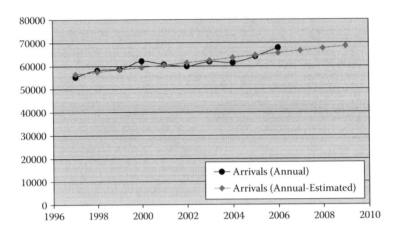

Figure 9.3   Annual visits to the York Hospital ED (1997–2006) and forecasted values (1997–2009).

regression model. Also in Table 9.1, b_1 = 1001.1, meaning that arrivals to the ED are growing at a rate of about 1,001 visits per year. The independent variable, *Year*, is statistically significant with a t-statistic of 5.65. (A reasonable rule of thumb is to conclude statistical significance when the absolute value of the *t*-statistic exceeds 2.) The SE_{reg} for this model (as given in the caption to Table 9.1, S = 1609.03) is 1,609 visits per year; that is, the difference between the actual annual visits and the number of visits estimated by the model is about 1,600 visits each year. This typical error (1,609) is about 2.6 percent of the average (60,947) annual arrivals, indicating good fit of the model.

Because these results suggest a reasonable model, we move to step 3—producing forecasts. To generate forecasts using trend-line regression, the last estimated value in the historical period (estimated visits in 2006 were 65,452) is added to the estimated number of visits each year (1,001). Using this procedure, the forecasted numbers of visits are: 66,453 in 2007; 67,454 in 2008; and 68,455 in 2009, calculations that are fully automated with regression software procedures. Figure 9.3 displays the historical values and the forecasts of annual visits, where we see reasonable cohesion between the values predicted by the trend-line regression model and the actual visits.

Regression packages produce prediction intervals that display potential forecast error. For example, the 95 percent prediction interval for the 2007 forecast of 66,453 visits is 61,959 to 70,947 (see Table 9.1). We'll discuss uses of these intervals later in the chapter.

Forecasting Monthly Visits for Tactical Planning: Staffing and Budgeting

To forecast monthly trends, we use the totals by month for the two most recent complete calendar years: 2005 and 2006. February was the slowest month with average arrivals of 5,064.5. The busiest month was December with 5,812 arrivals on average.

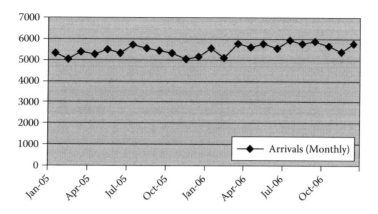

Figure 9.4   Monthly visits to the York Hospital ED, 2005–2006.

The forecasting goal is to produce monthly forecasts for 2007. As before, the initial step is examination of the time patterns. From Figure 9.4 we note that arrivals differ by month of the year and that arrivals are growing over this time period. A forecasting model should be chosen to capture both of these characteristics—something that regression can easily handle. The model is:

$$Arrivals\ (Monthly) = b_0 + b_1 Time + b_2 Jan + b_3 Feb + b_4 Mar + b_5 Apr + b_6 May$$
$$+ b_7 Jun + b_8 Jul + b_9 Aug + b_{10} Sep + b_{11} Oct + b_{12} Nov + \varepsilon.$$

In this model, *Time* is an integer-valued variable running from 1 to 24 (the total number of months in the data set). The *Time* variable serves the purpose of capturing the trend in the data; its coefficient, b_1, will be the estimate of the average monthly increase in arrivals. The remaining variables are monthly variables coded zero for that month and one for all other months. (As an example, the *Jan* variable will be one for all rows in the data set that are Januaries, and zero otherwise.) Note that the model does not contain a December monthly variable; even so, the relevant information for December is contained in the *y*-intercept, b_0. The remaining coefficients, b_2 through b_{12}, will measure the increase (or decrease) in arrivals that month relative to December.

The regression results are shown in Table 9.2. This model captures 93.4 percent of the variation in monthly arrivals as indicated by the R^2 statistic. The model, across all months, will have a typical error of about 98 arrivals (S = 97.96), which is quite good since the average number of monthly arrivals over this time period is 5,483. Arrivals are growing at a rate of about 25 more arrivals each month (the coefficient for *Time* in Table 9.2). We expect about 225 more arrivals in a typical January than in a typical December (see the coefficient for the *Jan* variable) and about 256 fewer arrivals in November than in December (*Nov*'s coefficient).

The numerical forecasts for 2007 are also shown in Table 9.2. This model predicts 5,523 arrivals for February 2007 (the slowest month); 6,271 arrivals

Table 9.2   Regression Results of Monthly Visits

Predictor	Coef	SE Coef	T	P
Constant	5015.75	91.64	54.74	0.000
Time	25.486	3.333	7.65	0.000
Jan	225.3	104.6	2.15	0.054
Feb	−155.1	103.5	−1.50	0.162
Mar	339.4	102.5	3.31	0.007
Apr	150.4	101.5	1.48	0.167
May	313.9	100.7	3.12	0.010
Jun	91.42	99.98	0.91	0.380
Jul	464.93	99.37	4.68	0.001
Aug	285.94	98.87	2.89	0.015
Sep	253.46	98.47	2.57	0.026
Oct	70.97	98.19	0.72	0.485
Nov	−255.51	98.02	−2.61	0.024
New Obs	Fit	SE Fit	95% CI	95% PI
1	5878.3	91.6	(5676.6, 6079.9)	(5583.0, 6173.5)
2	5523.3	91.6	(5321.6, 5724.9)	(5228.0, 5818.5)
3	6043.3	91.6	(5841.6, 6244.9)	(5748.0, 6338.5)
4	5879.8	91.6	(5678.1, 6081.4)	(5584.5, 6175.0)
5	6068.8	91.6	(5867.1, 6270.4)	(5773.5, 6364.0)
6	5871.8	91.6	(5670.1, 6073.4)	(5576.5, 6167.0)
7	6270.8	91.6	(6069.1, 6472.4)	(5975.5, 6566.0)
8	6117.3	91.6	(5915.6, 6318.9)	(5822.0, 6412.5)
9	6110.3	91.6	(5908.6, 6311.9)	(5815.0, 6405.5)
10	5953.3	91.6	(5751.6, 6154.9)	(5658.0, 6248.5)
11	5652.2	91.6	(5450.6, 5853.9)	(5357.0, 5947.5)
12	5933.2	91.6	(5731.6, 6134.9)	(5638.0, 6228.5)

Note: The regression equation is: Arrivals (Monthly) = 5016 + 25.5 Time + 225 Jan − 155 Feb + 339 Mar + 150 Apr + 314 May + 91 Jun + 465 Jul + 286 Aug + 253 Sep + 71.0 Oct − 256 Nov. S = 97.96; R-Sq = 93.4%; R-Sq(adj) = 86.2%.

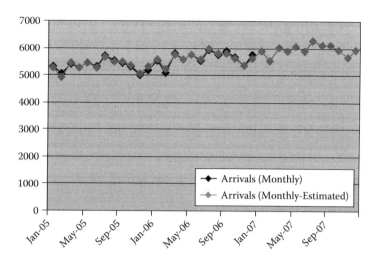

Figure 9.5   Monthly visits to the York Hospital ED (2005–2006) and forecasted values (2007).

for July 2007 (the busiest month); and ending the year with 5,933 arrivals in December 2007. Figure 9.5 displays the plot of the actual and predicted values, again indicating a close fit of the model to the data.

Forecasting Daily Visits for Operational Planning: Staffing and Scheduling

For staffing and scheduling, we would like to know differences in arrivals by day of the week. The forecasting objective is to derive daily estimates of arrivals for the first 10 days in January 2007 using daily historical data from CY2005–2006. Over the historical period, Sundays had the highest number of average arrivals (191), followed by Mondays (189) and Saturdays (181). Arrivals were lowest on average on Fridays (171).

Our data set contains 730 daily observations over two years—far too many to discern patterns from a time plot. Instead, Figure 9.6 displays daily patterns

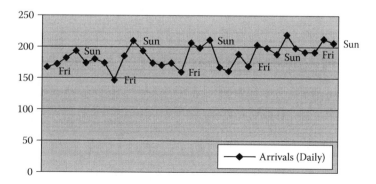

Figure 9.6   Daily visits to the York Hospital ED, December 2006.

for just December 2006, in which we see weekend peaks in arrivals and lower numbers of arrivals on Fridays. From our previous forecasting examples, we know that arrivals are increasing over time and that there is variation from month-to-month. Our daily forecasting model should also take these patterns into account. This requires a simple extension of the earlier monthly regression model in which variables are added to the model to account for daily variation:

$$Arrivals\ (Daily) = b_0 + b_1\ Time + b_2\ Jan + b_3\ Feb + b_4\ Mar + b_5\ Apr + b_6\ May \\ + b_7\ Jun + b_8\ Jul + b_9\ Aug + b_{10}\ Sep + b_{11}\ Oct + b_{12}\ Nov + b_{13}\ Mon \\ + b_{14}\ Tue + b_{15}\ Wed + b_{16}\ Thu + b_{17}\ Fri + b_{18}\ Sat + \varepsilon.$$

Here, for example, *Mon* is a variable whose values are one for days that are Mondays and zero otherwise. There is no Sunday variable because this day will be captured by the *y*-intercept. The coefficients for the weekday variables are interpreted as the typical amount by which that day's arrivals will be more or less than arrivals on a typical Sunday.

The regression results are shown in Table 9.3. The coefficient for *Time* indicates that arrivals are growing at a rate of about 0.03 more arrivals each day. Expect about 1.6 fewer arrivals on a typical Monday than a typical Sunday (*Mon*'s coefficient). Expect about 20 fewer arrivals on a typical Friday than a typical Sunday (*Fri*'s coefficient). The predicted number of arrivals for Monday, January 1, 2007 is 198, with 95% prediction interval of 171 to 225.

The regression model shown in Table 9.3 captures 34.4 percent of the variation in daily arrivals. This is quite a bit lower than the associated figures for the annual and monthly models, a result that is probably not surprising to those who work in EDs—variations from day to day are much more unpredictable than variations in monthly or annual aggregates. The regression model error is about 14 arrivals per day (see S in Table 9.3), which is 7 percent of the average daily arrivals of 180. Figure 9.7 shows the actual and estimated arrivals. The graph shows that the regression model picks up the general pattern in the daily data and that there are some notable differences between the actual number of arrivals and estimated arrivals in December 2006. We will have more to say about these results later in the chapter.

Forecasting Hourly Visits for Operational Planning: Scheduling

For identifying patterns in arrivals by hour of the day, we used the last full week in the 2003/04 fiscal year (June 20–26, 2004). Over this week, arrivals by hour were tabulated, resulting in 168 hourly observations in the data set. Arrivals averaged 7.3 per hour over this week. The hourly time plot shown in Figure 9.8 displays a classic sinusoidal pattern. *Fourier regression* is the form of regression

Table 9.3   Regression Results of Daily Visits

Predictor	Coef	SE Coef	T	P
Constant	173.250	2.585	67.02	0.000
Time	0.027297	0.002760	9.89	0.000
Jan	6.511	2.616	2.49	0.013
Feb	12.404	2.649	4.68	0.000
Mar	11.386	2.563	4.44	0.000
Apr	10.518	2.558	4.11	0.000
May	9.670	2.519	3.84	0.000
Jun	9.099	2.520	3.61	0.000
Jul	14.478	2.484	5.83	0.000
Aug	9.221	2.472	3.73	0.000
Sep	14.494	2.480	5.84	0.000
Oct	1.479	2.454	0.60	0.547
Nov	−2.564	2.470	−1.04	0.300
Mon	−1.640	1.885	−0.87	0.385
Tue	−12.980	1.886	−6.88	0.000
Wed	−14.712	1.887	−7.80	0.000
Thu	−17.790	1.887	−9.43	0.000
Fri	−20.128	1.886	−10.67	0.000
Sat	−9.767	1.881	−5.19	0.000

Predicted Values for New Observations (Jan. 1–10, 2007)

New Obs	Fit	SE Fit	95% CI	95% PI
1	198.076	2.573	(193.024, 203.127)	(170.852, 225.299)
2	186.763	2.586	(181.686, 191.839)	(159.535, 213.991)
3	185.058	2.599	(179.955, 190.161)	(157.825, 212.291)
4	182.007	2.600	(176.902, 187.113)	(154.774, 209.241)
5	179.696	2.602	(174.588, 184.805)	(152.462, 206.930)
6	190.086	2.593	(184.995, 195.177)	(162.855, 217.316)
7	199.880	2.578	(194.818, 204.941)	(172.654, 227.105)
8	198.267	2.584	(193.194, 203.340)	(171.040, 225.494)
9	186.954	2.597	(181.855, 192.052)	(159.722, 214.186)
10	185.249	2.610	(180.125, 190.374)	(158.012, 212.486)

Note: The regression equation is: Arrivals (Daily) = 173 + 0.0273 Time + 6.51 Jan + 12.4 Feb + 11.4 Mar + 10.5 Apr + 9.67 May + 9.10 Jun + 14.5 Jul + 9.22 Aug + 14.5 Sep + 1.48 Oct − 2.56 Nov − 1.64 Mon − 13.0 Tue − 14.7 Wed − 17.8 Thu − 20.1 Fri − 9.77 Sat. S = 13.6252; R-Sq = 34.4%; R-Sq(adj) = 32.8%.

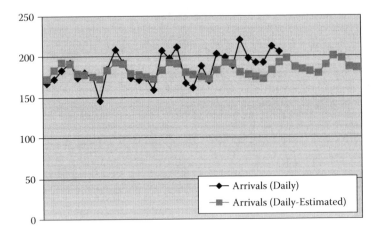

Figure 9.7   Daily visits to the York Hospital ED (December 2006) and forecasted values (January 1–10, 2007).

analysis capable of handling a wavelike pattern of this sort. The regression equation is:

$$Arrivals\ (Hourly) = b_0 + b_1 \sin(2\pi Time/24) + b_2 \cos(2\pi Time/24) + \varepsilon,$$

where sin and cos are sine and cosine functions that serve the purpose of producing the wave pattern. *Time* is an integer-valued counter variable running from 1 for the first hour in the data set and 168 for the last hour in the data set. In the equation, the division by 24 in the two independent variables defines the number of observations needed to complete one cycle (here, 24 hours in one day.)

The regression results are shown in Table 9.4. The model accounts for 47.4 percent of the variation in hourly arrivals. The typical error in any one hour is 2.7 arrivals. The sine and cosine independent variables are statistically

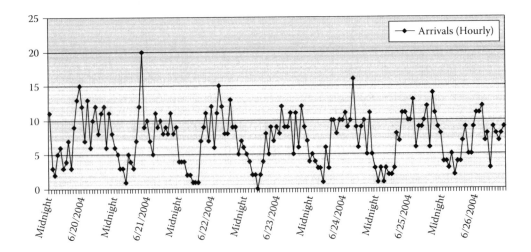

Figure 9.8   Hourly visits to the York Hospital ED, June 20–26, 2004.

Table 9.4   Regression Results of Hourly Visits

Predictor	Coef	SE Coef	T	P
Constant	7.2857	0.2056	35.44	0.000
sin(2PiTime/24)	−3.2743	0.2908	−11.26	0.000
cos(2PiTime/24)	−1.3624	0.2908	−4.69	0.000

Predicted Values for New Observations

New Obs	Fit	SE Fit	95% CI	95% PI
1	5.122	0.356	(4.419, 5.825)	(−0.186, 10.431)
2	4.469	0.356	(3.766, 5.172)	(−0.840, 9.777)
3	4.007	0.356	(3.304, 4.710)	(−1.301, 9.316)
4	3.769	0.356	(3.066, 4.472)	(−1.540, 9.077)
5	3.770	0.356	(3.067, 4.473)	(−1.538, 9.079)
6	4.011	0.356	(3.308, 4.715)	(−1.297, 9.320)
7	4.476	0.356	(3.772, 5.179)	(−0.833, 9.784)
8	5.131	0.356	(4.428, 5.834)	(−0.177, 10.440)
9	5.934	0.356	(5.231, 6.637)	(0.625, 11.242)
10	6.828	0.356	(6.125, 7.532)	(1.520, 12.137)
11	7.754	0.356	(7.051, 8.457)	(2.446, 13.063)
12	8.648	0.356	(7.945, 9.351)	(3.340, 13.957)
13	9.449	0.356	(8.746, 10.152)	(4.141, 14.758)
14	10.103	0.356	(9.400, 10.806)	(4.794, 15.411)
15	10.564	0.356	(9.861, 11.268)	(5.256, 15.873)
16	10.803	0.356	(10.099, 11.506)	(5.494, 16.111)
17	10.801	0.356	(10.098, 11.504)	(5.493, 16.110)
18	10.560	0.356	(9.857, 11.263)	(5.252, 15.869)
19	10.096	0.356	(9.393, 10.799)	(4.787, 15.404)
20	9.440	0.356	(8.737, 10.143)	(4.132, 14.749)
21	8.638	0.356	(7.934, 9.341)	(3.329, 13.946)
22	7.743	0.356	(7.040, 8.446)	(2.434, 13.051)
23	6.817	0.356	(6.114, 7.520)	(1.509, 12.126)
24	5.923	0.356	(5.220, 6.626)	(0.615, 11.232)

Note: The regression equation is: Arrivals (Hourly) = 7.29 − 3.27 sin(2PiTime/24) − 1.36 cos(2PiTime/24). S = 2.66492; R-Sq = 47.4%; R-Sq(adj) = 46.8%.

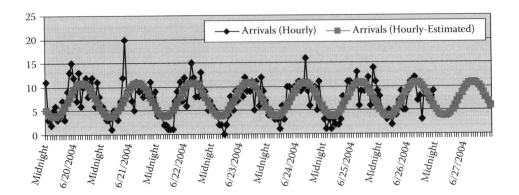

Figure 9.9   Hourly visits to the York Hospital ED (June 20–26, 2004) and forecasted values (June 27, 2004).

significant, since their t-ratios exceed 2 in absolute value. The forecasted values for June 27, 2004, are also displayed in Table 9.4. The first forecasted value is the hour beginning at midnight on June 27; expect about five arrivals then, with a slight decline until 5 a.m. when arrivals are estimated to be four. Peak arrivals of about ten per hour are predicted in the afternoons from 1 p.m. to 6 p.m., at which point arrivals slowly decline to about six arrivals per hour throughout the remainder of the day. Actual and forecasted hourly visits are shown in Figure 9.9.

Using Forecast Prediction Intervals

The annual, monthly, daily, and hourly forecasts shown in Tables 9.1, 9.2, 9.3, and 9.4 represent the regression model's best guess of arrivals at any point in time; they might be viewed as estimated *average* numbers of arrivals. Many service industries purposely choose not to use the average expected service level to make allocation decisions, since using average demand can be expected to leave them underallocated about half the time. Presumably this is pertinent to critical care delivery in emergency departments. Emergency department managers might wish to use the upper limits of the 95-percent prediction intervals shown in Tables 9.1, 9.2, 9.3, and 9.4. By doing so, they are more likely to have adequate resources during times of unexpectedly high demand, with the downside of having idle resources during unanticipated low demand. We particularly advocate using upper prediction intervals for those cases in which the regression model contains a lot of unexplained variance—in these data, the daily and hourly forecasts.

Discussion

The purpose of this chapter is to help ED medical directors make sense of their ED demand data and to show how they can use simple forecasting models to inform their strategic, tactical, and operational decision making. One statistical procedure, regression analysis, is shown to be versatile enough to handle a wide variety of forecasting needs, from long-term annual forecasts to short-term hourly forecasts. The data needed to conduct these analyses are routinely collected in EDs, in which arrivals are time-stamped and electronically recorded. Much of the effort to produce the forecasts involves organizing the raw data in such a way that it can be used in regression software packages.

Limitations

Forecasts will, of course, always be wrong. Even so, judicious use of forecasting models involves objective discovery and extrapolation of underlying patterns in data to assist in preparing for the uncertain future. Models also provide explicit numerical estimates of the potential size of forecast errors, which can be brought explicitly into the decision-making process. Thus, we advocate the use of forecasting models for ED managers provided some considerations are made.

Model-Specific Considerations

We used the York Hospital ED data to illustrate the power of regression models to handle a wide range of forecasting situations. Different settings might experience different arrival patterns than those shown in this chapter. Even so, regression analysis can easily handle most modeling situations that might arise in ED settings. Examples include the following:

- Annual, monthly, or hourly trends are not linear. The most common situation involves trends that increase (or decrease) at an increasing rate. In this case, the regression model should include an additional independent variable whose values are the square of the values in *Time* (for monthly or daily forecasts) or *Year* (for annual forecasts).
- Hourly arrivals have secondary peaks. For example, arrivals might peak during the afternoons, but display a notable secondary increase in late evenings. In this case, two additional independent variables can be added to the regression equation: $\sin(4\pi Time/24)$ and $\cos(4\pi Time/24)$.
- Daily arrivals are impacted by holidays. This situation is easy to handle using regression by adding additional zero/one independent variables to the model for different holidays.

Because these and other situations can be readily handled by regression analysis, ED managers need familiarity with only one statistical model to produce forecasts.

Data-Specific Considerations

The astute reader will note that we used different historical time periods depending on whether we were generating annual, monthly, daily, or hourly forecasts. For example, the historical period used for the annual forecasts was 1997 through 2006, but we used 2005–2006 to generate the monthly forecasts. What time periods, then, should be used to generate the regression forecasts? At least in part, the answer depends on the availability of data; for instance, we had no hourly historical data after 2004. Managers of relatively new emergency departments or those with established EDs that have just recently begun collecting usable data will be limited by the information available. For those with a richer historical data set, several rules of thumb can be used to select historical time periods. For annual forecasts, a decade's worth of data should be sufficient to establish a trend unless there has been a dramatic change in recent ED arrivals. For the monthly and daily forecasts, the historical data should be long enough so that each month or day is represented at least twice in the data set, implying, for example, at least two years of data for the monthly forecasts. Short-term hourly forecasts typically display no trend, so recent data that is representative of expected traffic should suffice. In all cases, though, forecasting projects require periodic updating of the historical data as new data becomes available. We recommend performing revisions at least once a year, and more often if ED personnel report notable changes in arrival patterns.

Software Considerations

Spreadsheets, such as Microsoft Excel, available to most ED managers can be used to undertake the initial preparation of the data. Spreadsheets can also handle the simpler procedures outlined in this chapter, such as annual and monthly forecasts. Regrettably, spreadsheets are limited in scope. For example, spreadsheets will not reliably handle the larger models required to produce daily forecasts. Some spreadsheets also have known computational problems that can produce incorrect forecasts. They can also require complicated behind-the-scenes manipulation of the data. For these reasons, we advocate the use of a statistical software package. Thankfully, almost all statistical software contains regression procedures and are relatively easy to use; software most likely to be found in hospital settings that conduct regression analysis include SAS, SPSS, and Minitab.

Acknowledgments

This presentation is based upon work supported by the National Science Foundation Grant No. 0323664. All opinions, findings, and conclusions or recommendations expressed in this chapter are those of the researchers and do not necessarily reflect the views of the National Science Foundation.

References

1. Akçali, Elif, Murray J. Côté, and Chin-I Lin, "A Network Flow Approach to Optimizing Hospital Bed Capacity Decisions." *Health Care Management Science*, 9, 4 (2006), 391–404.
2. Wright, P. Daniel, Kurt M. Bretthauer, and Murray J. Côté, "Reexamining the Nurse Scheduling Problem: Staffing Ratios and Nursing Shortages," *Decision Sciences*, 37, 1 (2006), 39–70.

Chapter 10

Improving Fairness in Nurse Scheduling:
Introducing a New Approach Using Auctions and Integer Programming Optimization

Melanie L. DeGrano

Introduction

As an industrial engineering student, I was aware that a number of operations research (management science) analytic toolsets in which I was being trained could benefit health care operations management decision makers. I have many friends who work within hospitals. I became aware through discussions with them, and via my own life experiences, that the creation of work schedules, obviously of great importance to frontline workers, is usually done manually, is very time intensive for managers/schedulers, and is often felt by the workers to lack fairness. Integer programming and optimization is a methodology routinely taught to industrial engineering students that lends itself to complex scheduling issues: the need to schedule staff in the context of multiple known constraints and then mathematically arrive at an optimal solution. I decided to apply what I had learned about integer programming and optimization in the classroom to improve fairness in nurse scheduling. Thus, I developed an auction (bidding) approach to antecede a traditional integer programming solution.

The United States is experiencing a substantial nursing shortage, projected to increase over the next two decades[1]. High turnover rates of nursing staff are a result of significant levels of job dissatisfaction; inflexible work schedules are a contributing factor to dissatisfaction[2]. Many hospitals have instituted self-scheduling in an attempt to both provide flexibility and increase job satisfaction for nurses.

In the self-scheduling approach, each nurse submits an individual schedule or request. A nurse manager then creates the base schedule for the care unit. In many hospital service units, the schedule is created manually after reviewing the requests with final approval and conflict resolution performed by the nurse manager. Manual scheduling and conflict resolution can take many hours, sometimes days, to complete. The individual preferences of staff may not be reflected in the resulting base schedule due to the difficulties inherent in manual scheduling and to direct conflicts.

Many computerized nurse scheduling heuristics and optimization algorithms have been proposed. Kellogg and Walczak[3] found that few such approaches have been accepted by practitioners and argued that there is a need for algorithms that accommodate the self-scheduling approach that currently predominates in practice.

The concept of an auction is not new in nurse scheduling. During the course of my initial research, I discovered that some hospitals were using auctions to fill vacant shifts. These hospitals allowed their nurses to bid on extra shifts (overtime) after base hours had already been scheduled to allow them to earn more money or to work a shift in a different department within their hospital to broaden their knowledge. The catch is that the nurses are bidding the hourly rate that they will be paid on the shift; in other words, the nurse willing to work the shift for the lowest pay wins[4–6]. I felt that the idea was novel and that it could be applied to base hours with some adjustments. To the best of my knowledge, auctions have not yet been used in practice to create the base schedule, because there is no built-in mechanism to ensure that hospital requirements are met. Such requirements include minimum time off between shifts, minimum and maximum hours worked per week, and coverage for each shift. Because of these constraints, a bid for a particular shift cannot be evaluated in isolation. A bid could be invalidated because it is inconsistent with other bids submitted by that individual or because honoring the bid could prevent generation of a feasible schedule for other nurses in the unit.

For my dissertation, I developed a new method for scheduling base hours for a nursing unit. The method starts by obtaining nurses' preferences for specific days and shifts, and works to build a schedule that accommodates those preferences while maintaining important hospital constraints. An auction is used to obtain preferences: nurses bid on work shifts and rest days using "points"; shifts are awarded to the highest bidders insofar as possible.

Literature Review

The literature reveals that some researchers have ignored nurses' preferences completely[7,8]. Others have developed a group preference rating for each shift by using perceived preferences[9], preferences for a particular shift pattern in a cyclic schedule[10], or aggregate preferences from survey[11]. A few researchers have attempted to incorporate individual nurse preferences, but they treat them as soft constraints, which can be violated[12,13].

In an attempt to provide nurses with more flexibility, "self-scheduling" was introduced[14–17]. This approach allows nurses to sign up for the shifts they want to work during each scheduling period, given predetermined coverage needs and rules defining acceptable schedules. Self-scheduling may involve negotiation among nurses in the unit. The nurse manager coordinates the scheduling, resolves conflicts, and produces the final schedule. Nurses' perceived control of scheduling is positively associated with job satisfaction[2]; thus, allowing nurses to schedule themselves can improve retention. Although self-scheduling provides more flexibility, it is time consuming. In addition, it can be very difficult to guarantee fairness, especially in cases where signing up for shifts is done on a first-come, first-served basis.

Recently, auctions have emerged as a method for scheduling overtime hours. Nurses bid on open shifts, with bids starting at a predefined maximum pay rate; shifts are awarded to the lowest bidder[4–6]. User reports indicate that the average winning bid is higher than the nurses' base rates[6,18]. Though some hospitals are concerned about this type of system[4], many hospitals have benefited from overtime shift auctions. Hospitals have experienced significant savings by reducing their use of temporary nurses from outside agencies (agency nurses are generally more expensive and may be less productive if they are not familiar with the hospital's routines). Nurses are more satisfied because they control how much overtime they work and their overtime pay rate. In some hospitals, nurses are permitted to bid for overtime work in other departments and thus can gain additional experience helpful for career advancement.

The overtime auctions seen in practice cannot be used for scheduling regular hours. Typically, nurses are contracted to work a specified number of base hours at a predetermined compensation rate; contract changes would be needed before any pay-based bidding system could be used. In addition, an auction alone cannot guarantee a schedule that meets coverage requirements and other hospital constraints. In the following section, I describe a combination of auctions and optimization to create a base schedule for a nursing unit.

Methods: General Discussion

It is beyond the scope of this chapter to discuss the mathematical specifics of the models and their derivation. The interested reader is referred to the author (mxd265@yahoo.com) for further information in this regard. I will next provide a high-level overview of the methodology that should be of interest to a regular, nonengineer hospital manager seeking to use new methods to improve current-day emergency department (ED) nurse scheduling practices.

This new scheduling process consists of two stages: an auction stage, in which nurses bid for their preferred shifts and the winners are selected; and a schedule completion stage, which assigns nurses to any vacant shifts. An auction can be set up in a variety of ways; I chose to use a sealed bid auction approach. A sealed bid auction is characterized by a single bidding round in which bidders do not see other individuals' bids and cannot update bids once they submit them[19]. A sealed bid auction fits well in this research because it is a simple and practical choice for nurses. The nurses on any unit can submit bids once and not have to worry about updating them. Furthermore, an approach based on sealed bid auction provides an easy transition and improvement upon the self-scheduling methodology that nurses and hospitals currently favor[3].

Once bidding is complete, winners are selected using an optimization model, which seeks to award shifts to the highest bidders while simultaneously meeting hospital requirements. After winners have been determined, the schedule completion stage uses a second optimization model to allocate the unfilled shifts to nurses who have not yet met their minimum hours. The stages are now explained in more detail.

Setting Up the Auction Stage

The schedule period for the nursing unit (e.g., one week, one month, etc.), the number of shifts per day, and the required coverage for each shift are determined before the auction takes place. Nurses are allocated a predetermined number of points to use for bidding. In the present iteration of the work, it is assumed that each nurse will have the same number of points. Note that in practice, however, nurse managers might consider providing senior nurses more points or awarding points to nurses on a performance-based system.

The auction stage consists of a bidding step followed by an award step. The bidding is flexible; in other words, nurses may split up their points for shifts however they like. Nurses make their selections and submit a bid package with their "on" and "off" shifts, as well as the number of points they have allocated to each. Each nurse submits a complete bid package before any awards are made. This bid package could be submitted on paper or theoretically using a Web interface. Because a sealed bid auction is used, only one bidding round takes place.

In the award step, bids are sorted in descending order with respect to the point value, and the highest bidders are selected as candidate winners. The number of candidate winners for "on" shifts is dictated by the staffing requirement for the particular shift; thus, if three nurses are needed, then there may be a first, second, and third place candidate winner. For "off" bids, the number of candidate winners is determined by the total number of nurses less the upper limit of requirements for a particular shift. For example, if there are eight nurses available and each shift can have no more than five working at a time, then the total "off" candidate winners in the auction will be three.

Creating the Optimization Model

The award step selects winners using an optimization model. The optimization model's constraints are specific to the particular hospital, since the schedule it generates must meet that hospital's requirements. The award step first checks the candidate winning bids to determine if a feasible schedule can be constructed if those candidates are selected as winners (awarded the shift). This is accomplished with the optimization model. If the candidate winning bids are feasible, the award step is complete and all candidates are awarded their shifts. If not, the model selects winners by maximizing the point value of all awarded bids. Any candidate winning bids that either violate hospital constraints or prevent construction of a feasible schedule will not be awarded. For example, if a nurse is a candidate winner of two consecutive 12-hour shifts, the model awards at most one of them. Also, if a nurse is a candidate winner of a shift but awarding it would cause another nurse to have insufficient rest time between shifts, the model will not award the shift.

Finally, the auction stage outputs a set of auction winners. These are the candidate winning bids that can be awarded while maintaining overall feasibility and that maximize the total bid points awarded.

The Schedule Completion Stage

The schedule completion stage of the model schedules additional shifts for nurses who have not met their working hour requirements by winning shifts in the auction. This stage guarantees that all shifts have adequate coverage and that the minimum nursing hours are satisfied for each nurse. The schedule completion stage also uses an optimization model. This second optimization model includes all the constraints used in the award model. Additional hard constraints require that wins from the auction stage are honored.

The assignment optimization model has a different objective function than was used in the award step. This objective function maximizes the total point value of assigned shifts, using only the bids that were not selected as candidate winners in the auction stage. Thus, it seeks a schedule in which losing bids are satisfied insofar as possible. For example, if a candidate winner cannot be awarded a shift in the auction stage, then another nurse will be assigned to that shift. The model will attempt to assign the highest bidding nonwinner, consistent with schedule feasibility.

It is possible to construct a single optimization model that both awards bids and completes the schedule. This can be accomplished by suitably weighting the candidate winning bids in the objective function. However, a two-stage approach is preferable, for several reasons. First, the nurse manager could review the winning bids and might choose to reject some of them. Second, a distinct auction stage can provide a basis for multiple auction rounds. Third, solving two smaller problems reduces computational requirements, although for the case study the reduction in solution time was minimal.

A Case Study

The auction-optimization method is now demonstrated using data from an ED at York Hospital in York, Pennsylvania. The case study included registered nurses (RNs) in the ED at York Hospital for the schedule period of March 18–April 14, 2007. The schedule for this time period had already been created using the hospital's current self-scheduling method, which it had been using since January 2007. Self-scheduling demands approximately 8 hours a week for the head nurse in charge of scheduling. Seven to eight weeks prior to the date a schedule is available, nurses are given blank scheduling sheets to fill in the shifts they prefer to work. According to the self-scheduling guidelines, nurses should sign up for all of their required hours. Nurses may also indicate up to four days they do not wish to work; any time off above four days in a week must be submitted as vacation time. Once the head nurse has all of the self-scheduling request forms, she manually enters them into the Automated Nurse Scheduling Office System (ANSOS), a system that reports a four-week schedule for a specified set of nurses. ANSOS was reported to have optimization capabilities[20]; however York Hospital does not have the optimization feature in its system. ANSOS is mainly used for reporting the schedule and determining the vacancies on each shift after the self-scheduling requests are submitted. Using the vacancies, the program reports the "Needs List," which is made available for nurses who would like to sign up for overtime. The schedule is then completed and posted three to four weeks in advance.

The study was performed to see how well the auction procedure would work using constraints at a real hospital. The self-scheduling requests from that schedule period were converted into bids, and the schedule produced using the auction-optimization method was compared to the official schedule. This approach avoided disruption of normal hospital operating procedures or placing extra demands on the nurses. In the following, the problem definition is presented, followed by implementation of the bidding step, the optimization models used for the award and assignment, and the overall algorithm implementation.

Problem (Constraints) Definition

At the time of this case study, York's ED had different types of nurses with various time commitments and experience levels. This single-schedule case study included registered nurses representing the following types:

- 28 full-time nurses who work 36 hours per week.
- 6 full-time nurses who work 40 hours per week.
- 6 part-time nurses; of these, 1 works 20 hours per week, 4 work 24 hours per week, and 1 works 28 hours per week.

Table 10.1   Nurse Requirement for 4-Hour Time Blocks

Time Period	Nurse Requirement
3 a.m.–7 a.m.	10
7 a.m.–11 a.m.	10
11 a.m.–3 p.m.	16
3 p.m.–7 p.m.	18
7 p.m.–11 p.m.	18
11 p.m.–3 a.m.	14

- 28 nurses under PRN contract. PRN stands for *pro re nata*, a Latin phrase meaning "occasionally" or "according to circumstances"[21]. These nurses are contracted to work either 16 or 24 hours per month, with certain requirements for weekend hours.
- 5 traveler nurses who work 36 hours per week during specified time periods.

The demand for staffing in the ED is measured in 4-hour time blocks, as certain portions of the day are busier than others. In addition, nurses can work shifts of differing length, including 4-, 8-, and 12-hour shifts. Table 10.1 shows the nurse requirement for each 4-hour time block.

Since the demand for nurses is based on a particular time period rather than shifts, it is necessary to determine the number of winners allowed per time period. This requires careful consideration of overlapping shifts. As an example, consider Table 10.2. In the table, there are six shifts that overlap the 3 a.m.–7 a.m. time period. A bid on any of those shifts would be competing for the same time slot.

Selecting candidate winners is based upon whether the bid is the highest in every time period it spans. For instance, a nurse who bids on the 3 a.m.–7 a.m.

Table 10.2   Example of Shifts Spanning Multiple Demand Periods

7 p.m.–11 p.m.	11 p.m.–3 a.m.	**3 a.m.–7 a.m.**	7 a.m.–11 a.m.	11 a.m.–3 p.m.
7 p.m.–7 a.m.				
	11 p.m.–11 a.m.			
	11 p.m.–7 a.m.			
		3 a.m.–3 p.m.		
		3 a.m.–11am		
		3 a.m.–7am		

Table 10.3   Example Requests for a Partial Schedule

	Sun 3/18	*Mon 3/19*	*Tues 3/20*	*Wed 3/21*	*Thurs 3/22*	*Fri 3/23*	*Sat 3/24*
Nurse 1	11a–7p				11a–11p	11a–7p	off

Table 10.4   Result of Translating a Request to a Bid in Example Problem

	Sun 3/18	*Mon 3/19*	*Tues 3/20*	*Wed 3/21*	*Thurs 3/22*	*Fri 3/23*	*Sat 3/24*
Nurse 1	15				23	15	47

shift and is the top bidder during all six time slots is a candidate winner. If the nurse is not the top bidder for each of the spanning slots but ranks high enough to fall within the number of winners allowed per slot, the bid is considered to be a candidate winner. In this example, the bid would need to be at least in 10th place since 10 is the minimum nurse requirement for shifts that span this time slot. Note that nurses only place one bid for a shift; their one bid amount will be used to compare to any other bidder whose shift spans a common time slot.

The number of winners allowed for "off" or rest days must also be specified. After examining York's schedule the number of winners was set to 15 for Saturdays and Sundays and 5 for weekdays.

Although active bidding was not performed with the RNs, the study was completed by using the self-scheduling requests. Since active bidding could not be done at this time, the bids were inferred from the self-scheduling requests. As an example, consider the partial schedule request shown in Table 10.3. This particular nurse requested three working shifts and one day off. To translate this request into a bid, each bid carried a weight in proportion to shift length, and "off" bids are weighted more heavily than "on" bids. Specifically, weights of 1 (4-hour shifts), 2 (8-hour shifts), 3 (12-hour shifts), and 6 (days off) were used. These weights were normalized and converted to bid points. The example of Table 10.3, assuming a total of 100 points for the week, results in the bids shown in Table 10.4.

York hospital creates schedules every four weeks, so the self-scheduling requests covered a 28-day time period. For this experiment, each nurse had 400 points for bidding over the period, and bids were calculated as described earlier. This approach was used to translate schedule requests that had already been submitted into bids for the award step. Note that in active bidding, nurses can make their bids however they want and would not have to follow any particular rule regarding allocation of points based on shift length.

Optimization Models

Integer programming optimization models are used for the award step of the auction and for the schedule completion stage. The optimization models must be configured to match a particular hospital's work rules, employee contracts, and other constraints or preferences. The hospital constraints at York Hospital are derived from hospital needs as well as considerations for nurses' health and well-being. Without fully presenting the equations, the following constraints were included in the case study:

- Satisfy daily staff requirements. Each shift must be covered by the minimum required number of nurses.
- Minimum rest time between shifts. The minimum rest time between shifts is 8 hours.
- Min/max working days per schedule. Each nurse has a contractual number of days required to work per monthly schedule.
- PRN 0: Nurses under PRN 0 designation must work 16 hours per month.
- PRN 1: Nurses under PRN 1 designation must work 24 hours per month, of which 8 hours must be on a weekend.
- PRN 3: Nurses under PRN 3 designation must work 24 hours every other weekend.
- PRN 3A: Nurses under PRN 3A designation must work 24 hours, three out of four weekends.
- PRN 4: Nurses under PRN 4 designation must work two 12-hour shifts every weekend.
- Monday/Friday constraint. Every nurse except PRN nurses must work at least two Mondays and/or Fridays in a month.

In addition, the constraints also had to account for a nurse shortage. At the time of the study, the ED had approximately 11.1 full-time equivalent (FTE) nurses. Since it is known that the emergency department is understaffed, there will not be enough nurses to meet coverage restrictions. To combat this issue, a dummy variable is introduced for each slot on each day that picks up the slack on the time slots that cannot fulfill the requirements. Thus, when the model is complete, the dummy variable represents the number of nurses still needed on a particular four-hour time slot. This will be used to determine the blocks of time that are suitable for any fill-in agency nurses or overtime sign-ups.

Other constraint adjustments had to be included in the model. Nurses often have mandatory education days or "project" days in which they are required to be at the hospital but are unavailable to care for patients. In most cases, the nurses will be on the schedule to work a total of 8 hours. These meetings are counted in their weekly hours but the nurses are not counted toward the staff requirement in the numbers for primary care.

Paid time off (PTO) may also be requested while bidding for the schedule. PTO includes vacation days or time that has accrued according to hours worked. Nurses who would like to use PTO will not have to use points to bid for it—it will automatically be considered a day off. Requests for days off which are not based on PTO must be done as bids. Similar to project and education days previously described, the 8 hours would be counted toward the nurses' weekly time commitments.

Case Study Results

The model contains 29,344 variables and 32,892 constraints, and is generated automatically. A program was developed to read the bids, select the candidate winners, generate the formulation, and call up an optimization solver. Determining the candidate winners and generating the formulation took 2.073 seconds. The award stage took 2 minutes and 55 seconds, and the schedule completion stage took 5.74 seconds. LINGO was used for optimization, and the software was run on an Intel Core 2 Duo processor T7200 (2GHz, 1 GB RAM). Altogether, the methodology required slightly more than 3 minutes of CPU time to generate a schedule, a significant time savings as compared to the manual method currently in use at York Hospital.

As evident in Table 10.5, the two methods are comparable in terms of percentage of requests fulfilled, but the auction-optimization model performed slightly better for "on" bids. The manual method awarded more "off" requests; however, after further investigation, it was found that the only losing "off" bids in the auction-optimization model were attributed to a traveler nurse who was ending a contract. This particular traveler nurse had written an X on his request form, which was meant to represent an end in contract but was mistakenly read as an "off" bid during the bid translation. Thus, four of the "off" bids that were not granted to the traveler nurse were actually days he was not supposed to be included on the schedule. When the constraints in the model were altered to reflect the actual situation, the unfulfilled "off" bids were avoided. Thus, the methods are equal in terms of awarding "off" shifts for this schedule. I chose to present this issue rather than correct it in the table to bring attention to such issues that may arise in practice. For implementation to be successful, nurse managers must be able to input any changes to the constraints on the front end before the model is run each scheduling period.

Table 10.5 Comparison of Overall Success

Request Type	% Requests Fulfilled Self-Scheduling	% Requests Fulfilled Auction-Optimization Model
"On" requests	90.48%	98.27%
"Off" requests	100%	95.51%

This study has demonstrated that the auction-optimization approach can capture both realistic hospital constraints and individual preferences, and can use them to generate a good schedule. The schedule is comparable to one generated by an experienced nurse manager. It took approximately 3 minutes to produce the schedule once the bids were input, whereas the current self-scheduling process demands approximately 8 hours per week of the head nurse's time per schedule.

An advantage of the auction-optimization approach is its similarity to self-scheduling: the bidding stage is very similar to the request submission process already in place. The only difference is that nurses will submit point values with their shift requests to reflect their strength of preference. Optionally, nurses could be allowed to bid on their strongest preferences rather than specify all of their working hours as with self-scheduling. If they bid on fewer hours than required, the assignment model would add shifts up to their required hours.

It should be noted that the emergency department at York Hospital is understaffed. Deficits are filled by allowing nurses to sign up for overtime hours or by allowing agency nurses to pick up shifts. If the hospital had adequate staffing, there could be more competition for shifts or rest days, and it is possible that the win percentages would be lower.

Conclusions

Unlike other scheduling methods in the literature, this auction-optimization approach directly accommodates the preferences of individual nurses. Having more influence on the scheduling process has been shown to promote feelings of autonomy and lead to increased job satisfaction. The auction-optimization method improves upon self-scheduling by allowing nurses to express their strength of preference through the amounts that they bid.

The results from applying the auction-optimization model to the emergency department at York Hospital as an off-line case study are very encouraging. Most nurse requests were fulfilled, and the schedule was generated in a reasonable amount of computer time. It should be stressed that the shortage of nurses makes it easier to fulfill bid requests. Simulation experiments show that win percentages are high, even with adequate staff levels. Note that in the current health care environment, nurse shortages are quite common, and therefore the case study results represent today's reality.

Acknowledgments

I would like to extend a heartfelt thanks to D.J. Medeiros for all of the knowledge and advice she has provided over the years. Dave Eitel and Blythe Stover-Baker from York Hospital are appreciated for their enthusiastic support during the development of the research, especially for contributing data so that the research could be applied to a real world situation.

References

1. Bureau of Health Professions (2004) What is behind HRSA's projected supply, demand, and shortage of registered nurses. Retrieved June 2008 from http://bhpr. hrsa.gov/healthworkforce/reports/behindrnprojections/index.htm.
2. Sagie A, Krausz M (2003) What aspects of the job have most effect on nurses? *Human Resource Management Journal* 13:46–62.
3. Kellogg D, Walczak S (2007) Nurse scheduling: From academia to implementation or not? *Interfaces* 37(4):355–369.
4. Koeppel D (2004) Nurses bid with their pay in auctions for extra work. *New York Times*, June 6.
5. Miller A (2004) Nursing shifts up for bid: Riverdale hospital to use Web to match RNs and extra work. *Atlanta Journal–Constitution*, August 13, E1.
6. Sidime A (2005) Bidding for work. *Knight Ridder Tribune Business News*, February 28.
7. Warner D, Prawda J (1972) A mathematical programming model for scheduling personnel in a hospital. *Management Science* 19(4):411–422.
8. Ferland J, Berrada I, Nabli I, Ahoid B, Michelon P, Gascon V, Gagne E (2001) Generalized assignment type goal programming problem: Application to nurse scheduling. *Journal of Heuristics* 7:391–413.
9. Abernathy W, Baloff N, Hershey J, Wandel S (1973) A three-stage manpower planning and scheduling model: A service-sector example. *Operations Research* 21(3):693–711.
10. Dowsland K, Thompson J (2000) Solving a nurse scheduling problem with knapsacks, networks and tabu search. *Journal of the Operational Research Society* 51:825–833.
11. Azaiez M, Al Sharif S (2005) A 0-1 goal programming model for nurse scheduling. *Computers & Operations Research* 32:491–507.
12. Berrada I, Ferland J, Michelon P (1996) A multi-objective approach to nurse scheduling with both hard and soft constraints. *Socio-Economic Planning* Science 30:183–193.
13. Miller H, Rath G, Pierskalla W (1976) Nurse scheduling using mathematical programming. *Operations Research*, 24:857–870.
14. Griesmer H (1993) Self-scheduling turned us into a winning team. *RN* 56(12):21–23.
15. Miller M (1984) Implementing self-scheduling. *Journal of Nursing Administration* 14:33–36.
16. Ringl K, Dotson L (1989) Self-scheduling for professional nurses. *Nursing Management* 20:42–44.
17. Silvestro R, Silvestro C (2000) An evaluation of nurse rostering practices in the National Health Service. *Journal of Advanced Nursing* 32:525–535.
18. Lawrence S (2004) System lets nurses bid for shifts. Retrieved September 2006 from http://www.eweek.com/article2/0,1895,1666200,00.asp.

19. Klemperer P (1999) Auction theory: A guide to the literature. *Journal of Economic Surveys* 13:227–286.
20. Warner M, Keller B, Martel S (1991) Automated nurse scheduling. *Journal of the Society for Health Systems* 2(2):66–80.
21. The Free Online Medical Dictionary (2007) p.r.n. Retrieved 2007 from http://medical-dictionary.thefreedictionary.com/p.r.n.

Chapter 11

Establishing Engineered Nurse Staffing Requirements in the Emergency Department

Frank Overfelt

Purpose of Engineered Staffing Ratios

The purpose of establishing engineered nurse staffing requirements in any area of nursing, including the emergency department (ED), is to ensure that the right resources (nurses) are in the right place (various locations throughout the emergency department) at the right times (covering all 24 hours of operation, 7 days a week). Implied in the foregoing statement is the right skill mix (right resources) of registered nurses, emergency medical technicians, unit secretaries, transporters, and the like.

To establish the appropriate staffing requirements the following ingredients must be identified and quantified:

- The arrival rate of patients by hour of day by day of week, by season, if necessary
- The various types of patients seen historically in the department (their acuity), ranging from heavy intense trauma cases to the less urgent types
- The respective service times for each step in the process that the patient will encounter
  - Quick registration
  - Triage
  - Nurse assessment
  - Physician assessment
  - Ancillary testing by exam, test, procedure

- The respective treatment profiles by presenting complaint
  - TPR
  - Assessments
  - Preparation for procedure
  - Medication administration
  - Transportation
- All other components of care

Arrival Rate of Patients

Historical information on the arrival patterns of patients by hour of day by day of week is essential information to have in order to place the correct number of staff at those times when the patient volume dictates. Even better information is to be able to compile information on patients within the system by hour of day by day of week. This latter concept takes into account not only the arrival rate of patients, but their length of stay as well. Most electronic tracking systems have the capability to provide both the arrival rate of patients by hour of day by day of week, as well as the number of patients in department by hour of day by day of week. As with simulation, this information is essential for developing models for managing patient flow.

Acuity of Patients

No two patients are totally alike. To assume that a patient is a patient (using predetermined fixed ratios) will provide flawed information relative to the staffing of the emergency department. Essential to distinguishing one patient from another, as far as treatment requirements are concerned, requires the presence of a patient acuity (presenting problem patient classification) system. Dr. David Eitel has codeveloped a presenting problem patient acuity system for the emergency department, called the Emergency Severity Index (ESI; www.ahrq.gov/research/esi).

The intent of a patient acuity system is to put homogeneous patients into similar groupings based upon the potential consumption of resources required to provide care for those patients. One can better evaluate the staffing requirements for an emergency department when the consumption of resources by acuity grouping is known.

Besides Eitel's grouping process, the Emergency Nurses Association also provides an acuity grouping methodology (www.ena.org).

Benefits to an Acuity System

Acuity systems provide the following benefits to emergency department management:

1. **A more precise measurement of workload requirements.** Rather than use one fixed ratio or composite HPV (hours per patient visit) for all patients, a number of varying ratios or HPV should be developed by acuity level.
2. **A foundation for nursing labor charges in the emergency department.** Using an acuity system enables the hospital to have varying charge levels based upon the intensity of nursing services being provided.
3. **Project a more accurate estimation for labor budgeting purposes.** Depending upon the variation and frequency of patients by acuity level, a more mix-sensitive-based budgeting system can be developed and historical trends can be monitored.
4. **Tracking acuity trends** will also assist management in identifying other resource consumptions: number of casts, imaging exams, inpatient admissions, and the like.

To illustrate what type of impact an acuity system can have on staffing, assume the following information:

- Total annual patient visits: 100,000
- An overall composite 3.25 hours per patient visit as one alternative
- A more mix-sensitive approach as the second alternative:
  1% level I visits, 1.84 HPV
  26% level II visits, 2.12 HPV
  36% level III visits, 3.15 HPV
  27% level IV visits, 5.14 HPV
  10% level V visits, 7.86 HPV

If those 100,000 visits are broken into the five categories or acuity levels, then the following results:

Level I: 1,000 visits times 1.84 HPV = 1,840 annual hours worked
Level II: 26,000 visits times 2.12 HPV = 55,120 annual hours worked
Level III: 36,000 visits times 3.15 HPV = 113,400 annual hours worked
Level IV: 27,000 visits times 5.14 HPV = 138,780 annual hours
Level V: 10,000 visits times 7.86 HPV = 78,600 annual hours
Total annual hours: 387,740

Compare this acuity-mixed result of 387,740 productive annual hours with the alternative of simply multiplying 100,000 with a benchmark 3.25 HPV, which equals 325,000 annual hours.

A variance of 62,740 hours results from this comparison. In full-time equivalent (FTE) terminology that equates to 30.16 FTEs. That variance indicates that the department could be understaffed by 30.16 FTEs.

Service Times

The various time standards (hours per patient visit) used in the aforementioned illustration are examples of the respective service times one could use to determine staffing. Service times would not include wait time. Components of these service time examples would include direct care, indirect care, and routine care:

Direct patient care
- Time for quick registration
- Time for triage
- Time to escort to room
- Nurse assessment
- Family interactions
- Nurse assist with procedure (if required)
- Nurse present with physician (if required)
- Escort to imaging (if required)
- Nurse discharge instructions
- Nurse transport to floor (if required)
- Nurse other

Indirect patient care
- Phone calls
- Computer interactions
- Discussion with peers
- Retrieval of medications
- Retrieval of supplies
- Clean up rooms
- Set up rooms
- Use of pneumatic tubes
- Other similar activities

Routine activities
- Shift reporting
- Narcotic counts
- Crash cart checks
- Other similar activities

Service times by acuity level times volumes of activities by acuity level equal the required productive hours.

The skill mix of the individuals performing these activities also needs to be taken into account. Some of the aforementioned activities can be performed by registered nurses (RNs) only, whereas others could be delegated to emergency medical technicians (EMTs) or clinical care assistants. Unit secretaries serve an important function in the emergency department, processing orders, preparing paperwork, and contributing to the continuity of care in the department.

Treatment Profiles

Once service times have been established for all the activities, then treatment profiles by acuity levels can be developed. These treatment profiles are simply profiles on the types of activities performed for each acuity level of patient. The frequency with which each task in a treatment profile is performed needs to be determined.

Factors Affecting the Expenditure of Time in the Emergency Department

Because no two emergency departments are totally alike, the nuances of each department must be taken into account. These nuances can be grouped into (1) ancillary support, (2) technological support, (3) ergonomic issues, (4) bed turnover, and (5) staff turnover.

1. Ancillary support
   a. What type of support do other departments provide the emergency department?
      i. Does imaging retrieve and return ED patients for all exams, some exams, or no exams?
      ii. Is there a respiratory therapist in the ED 24/7?
      iii. Does transport take patients to inpatient rooms?
      iv. What support does environmental services provide the ED?
      v. Are supplies replenished by materials management?
   b. How are these departments notified of ED service requirements?
      i. Paged?
      ii. Via computer?
      iii. Order entry?
2. Technological support
   a. Does the ED utilize electronic medical records and what impact does this have on the recording and acquisition of data?
   b. What type of "tracking" system does the department utilize? What information is available on the tracking system that affects the patient flow of the department?
   c. Is there an electronic medication dispensing system in use in the ED?
   d. Is there an electronic supply dispensing system in the ED?

    e. Does the department utilize a "passive" tracking system? (Basically this is a system that requires the staff and patient to be outfitted with a device that is tied to a radio-frequency identification [RFID] tag to automatically track the location of each patient or staff member.)

  3. Ergonomic factors

    a. Is there an urgent care area of the ED? What are the hours of operations of the urgent care center? Is this area used as backup for the ED during busier times? Does it have its own nursing station and accoutrements?

    b. What is the proximity of the ED to imaging? Does the ED have its own CT (computed tomography) or chest x-ray machines?

    c. Where is the location of the medication dispensing station, supply dispensing station, pneumatic tube system (and what labs can be sent via pneumatic tube), linen supply, and so forth?

    d. Is there a dedicated cast room? Who staffs this cast room (ortho techs, ED techs) and what hours of operation does it have?

  4. Bed Turnover

    a. How admissions to the Emergency Department are there?

    b. How long is the length of stay of patients in the ED?

    c. What causes delays in getting patients into beds?

    d. What are the admitting practices of the individual ED physicians?

      i. Do they wait until the end of a shift to release the patients?

      ii. How are admissions coordinated between the ED physician, ED Nurses and House Supervision

    e. Is there a bed control system in place in the hospital?

  5. Staff Turnover

    a. What is the turnover rate of Nurses in the Emergency Department?

    b. What contributes to the turnover rate?

    c. What can be done to resolve issues contributing to turnover of staff?

    d. What team building programs are in place?

    e. What has been done to improve communications among the nurses and the physicians? Are proper expectations communicated?

    f. During a given shift is there a high turnover of staff built in to accommodate hourly arrival patterns? How are reports among departing and arriving nurses handled?

Methodologies for Developing Engineered Nurse Staffing Requirements

A number of variations on how to develop engineered staffing requirements in the emergency department will be presented in this section. Each variation or option has its benefits and drawbacks.

Detailed Zero-Based Staffing

The most detailed, and therefore the most accurate, but also the most costly approach is applying a zero-based approach to setting staffing requirements. This approach utilizes a number of detailed data collection documents, some of which must be completed by the staff. In a methodology developed by the Delta Healthcare Consulting Group, four data collection documents are deployed to capture detailed information. These documents are:

Direct care document—This document is a mirror image of what is documented in the patient's chart or electronic medical record, and includes the frequencies of all activities, procedures, and the like performed by nurses at the patient's bedside. Examples of these activities include: vital signs, assessments, procedures, IV starts, and so forth. Typically a nurse chart extractor (not part of daily staffing) would complete this form.

Nondocumented direct care document (bedside sheet)—This document contains those activities or tasks that are also performed at the patient bedside, but are not documented in the patient's chart. Examples of these activities include: provide nourishments, assist to commode, repositioning, emotional and teaching support for the patient and family, and the like. The nurse or EMT assigned to the patient would be responsible for recording frequency of tasks on this form. Data are collected according to skill mix performing the task.

Indirect data collection document—This document could take many forms. One of the forms would be designed to collect all the activities that would be performed at the nurses' station. Another variation of the form would be to collect errands occurring off the unit. Other forms could be used to collect approaches to the medication dispensing, supply dispensing, use of the pneumatic tube, and the like. Examples of tasks collected on this document include phone calls in and out, interactions among staff members and among physicians, computer interactions, and the like. Again, data are collected by skill mix.

Routine activities data collection document—The routine activities collection only requires having the nurse manager describe the number of routine activities and their respective frequencies and times. No one needs to collect data to complete this document. Examples of activities found on this sheet include: crash cart check, rounds, shift reporting, charge nurse–to–charge nurse report, and the like.

Use of Predetermined Treatment Profiles

Utilizing treatment profiles by acuity level from other facilities, modifications can be made and customized to fit the uniqueness of the studied facility. The treatment profiles have been formulated from the detailed data collection described earlier. This alternative requires far less dedication.

Work Sampling

A widely used approach to establishing staffing requirements is to utilize third-party consultants to observe staff members every 10 to 15 minutes throughout the day. Work sampling focuses on the staff rather than on the patient (zero-based staffing and treatment profiles focus on the patient). Work sampling has the added advantage that trained observers can identify process and workload improvements while they are sampling. Typically a sampling period is one 24-hour period, which may be done 8 hours at a time. Work sampling is a good technique to validate the more detailed data collection process.

Conclusion

Engineering nurse staffing requirements is a far superior approach to the legislated mandatory approach of fixed patient ratios, which does not take into account the variability of layout and design of each emergency department. It does not account for varying levels of support from ancillary departments or for the varying types of patients seen in the ED. The engineered approach takes into account the varying types of patients seen in the department. "A patient is not a patient" is the concept underlying the engineered staffing approach.

Chapter 12

Patient Safety Organizations:
*A New Paradigm in Quality Management
and Communication Systems in Health Care*

Douglas B. Dotan

Becoming a Learning Organization

> An estimated 2.2 million people have experienced medical error personally or with their families, according to the Commonwealth Fund (2002).

In every human endeavor, successful outcomes begin with a good plan and design. Good design requires innovative thinking and the ability to learn from successful outcomes. Unfortunately, more often than not, we wait to learn from mistakes and failures, particularly in high-risk and complex organizations. However, learning in most organizations is limited by internal and external, perceived and real communication barriers. Hence, these organizations are continually challenged with the need to vastly improve operations, safety, and outcomes. In today's world of 24-hour news coverage and instant messaging, operational risks (e.g., collapse of construction cranes, collisions on the runway, accidental release of toxic chemicals, product recalls, nosocomial infections, overdoses of heparin, and wrong-site surgery) that result in injury and fatality are magnified many fold in news media.

The health care sector is a prime example of a modern high-risk and complex organization. New surgical procedures, medical treatments, and therapies coupled with the latest breakthroughs in technology and medicines have contributed to the $2.1 trillion health care sector in the United States. It is the most expensive and advanced health care system in the world. Yet, compared to other industrialized nations, our health care system consistently ranks near the bottom in operational outcomes for health care organizations and in health outcomes for customers.

Experts are urging us to look at our health care system and reexamine the entire design, particularly in the area of communicating safety issues and learning from it. The challenge is to identify the issue and to provide the right solution to the need. In 2000, the Institute of Medicine (IOM) study *To Err is Human* recommended the Department of Health and Human Services (DHHS) design a national "quality organization" to protect information provided by caregivers to be used for patient safety reporting and systems improvement.

A learning organization is one that is successful at acquiring, cultivating, and applying knowledge that can be used to help it continually adapt to change (Greenberg and Baron, 2000). Whether they want to or not, all organizations change; some do it more effectively than others. Examples of industries that continually adapt to change include commercial aviation, petrochemical, and nuclear power. Ford Motor Company, Toyota, General Electric, Motorola, Wal-Mart, and Xerox are often cited as organizational leaders for innovation and improvement. Can hospitals become learning organizations and improve health care quality and patient safety?

The epitome of learning involves gathering the right data, processing them into usable information, and transforming information into knowledge (Dotan, 2002, 2004). All successful organizations that continually learn and adapt to forces in their environment have created the ability and capacity to build knowledge necessary to stay ahead of the competition and for survival. It is expected that learning organizations achieve their goals by building problem-solving teams and communities, and empowering staff to be innovative (Smith, 1995). Concomitantly, these organizations already have created the environment and culture for quality and safety, which foster team building, innovation, learning, and, most of all, open communication throughout the organization.

A National Patient Safety System from the Grassroots

> A quarter of the U.S. population, more than 45 million, are reported to be uninsured.

Unlike other countries, such as Great Britain, Germany, France, and Canada, with a socialized health care system and universal health coverage, we lack the organization and leadership at the national level to build a national health care safety system. As inherent to our inventive and pragmatic nature, great social and political movements often evolve from grassroots origins. Health care is not different. A critical mass is quickly building among concerned patients and families along with frustrated health care providers and third-party payers who are demanding drastic changes in the health care system beyond cost containment, equitable access, and affordability. Welcome to the dawn of the "patient-driven" or the "customer-demand" health care system.

Overall health care spending is expected to reach $4.3 trillion by 2017, rising from $7,026 a person to $13,101 a person by 2017.

Efforts to design and implement a national health care safety system as a way to improve health care quality and patient safety began more than 20 years ago, and probably much earlier. Driven by the growing demand to contain health care cost, serious discussion about a national health care plan and implementation was shared only in esoteric political and medical circles. Only recently have patients and other stakeholders been included in the talks and strategy for a true "patient-centered" health care system.

Following *To Err is Human,* the IOM published *Crossing the Quality Chasm: A New Health System for the 21st Century* (2001) with six specific aims and recommendations to improve health care from the perspective of the patient's experience:

1. Safety—Patients should not be harmed by the care that is intended to help them. Patient safety is freedom from accidental injury.
2. Effectiveness—Apply systematically acquired evidence to determine whether an intervention, such as a test or therapy, produces better outcomes. Provide services based on scientific knowledge to all who could benefit (avoid underuse) and refrain from providing services to those not likely to benefit (avoid overuse).
3. Patient-centeredness—Focus on the patient's experiences of illness and health care and on the systems that work or fail to work to meet individual patient's needs. Provide care that is respectful of and responsive to individual patient preferences, needs, and ensures that patient values guide all clinical decisions.
4. Timeliness—Reduce wait times and sometimes harmful delays for both those who receive and those who give care. Reduce administration or production costs.
5. Efficiency—Avoid waste, including waste of equipment, supplies, ideas, and energy.
6. Equity—Continually reduce the burden of illness, injury, and disability, and improve the health and functionality of people.

Many health care organizations are still struggling to meet all six aims of the IOM or finding difficulty in sustaining their progress and achievements in quality and safety. Although the operational goals have been formulated, organizational capacity in health care, especially to acquire the right information and build knowledge over time, is very limited. Therefore, most health care organizations will continue to struggle in learning and changing. The exceptions are those recognized for high achievements in quality by the Baldrige Awards, state awards, and other quality awards because success begets success. The number of health care institutions applying for quality awards is steadily increasing. These outstanding hospitals openly share their insights and best practices. Moreover, they strive to continually improve.

The Patient Safety and Quality Improvement Act of 2005

After being reviewed and passed by the U.S. Congress and Senate, the Patient Safety and Quality Improvement Act was signed into federal law on July 29, 2005 (Agency for Healthcare Research and Quality [AHRQ], 2008). To address the growing concern about patient safety by improving voluntary and confidential reporting of medical adverse events, this act demonstrates for the first time the federal government's commitment to create a system for the purpose of collecting, codifying, aggregating, and analyzing patient safety information. Patient safety organizations (PSOs) are the nodal points of this patient safety system that are to be set up independently to remove any fear of discovery of peer deliberations, medical malpractice litigation, and disciplinary actions for the person communicating concerns. All information will be treated confidentially and protected by a federal legal privilege. Additionally, the use of the information in criminal, civil, and administrative proceedings is limited. A violation of confidentiality or privilege protections can reach $10,000, enforced by the Office of Civil Rights of the DHHS (Clancy, 2008).

Despite the lack of federal funding, the Patient Safety Act defines the specific role of the PSO to conduct patient safety activities and evaluations. Such activities that involve developing and reporting patient safety information under a uniform set of federal protection to the PSO are known as the patient safety work product (PSWP). The process of internal deliberations between a provider and the PSO defines the patient safety evaluation system (PSES). Together the PSWP and PSES provide the mechanism to develop a more comprehensive organization and structure to collect and analyze patient safety information. Ultimately, the act requires the creation of a repository or clearinghouse of information called the Network of Patient Safety Databases (NPSD) to aggregate, archive, and share knowledge among providers, various PSOs, networks of PSOs, and stakeholders, such as DHHS and the Center for Medicare.

The Patient Safety Act specifies that PSOs are to work with more than one provider in a network. Public or private, profit or not-for-profit hospitals and hospital systems can be eligible to become PSOs. Insurance companies and their affiliates, as well as any entity with regulatory or accreditation authority over providers, however, are not eligible as PSOs.

Lessons Learned in Other Industries

A wise person learns from his mistakes; a wiser person learns from others' mistakes. For high-risk industries—particularly ones dealing with potential catastrophic outcomes with loss of properties, lives, and public trust—the latter learning option is preferred. Slowly we are becoming a society that strives to achieve high reliability, zero defects, and near-asymptotic perfection in operation and safety.

Organizations today are faced with the competition to maintain the lead by learning and implementing new ideas to continue their business of delivering goods and services. The only apparent change is that this competition has grown to the point that trial-and-error learning is no longer possible, feasible, or even ethical. Therefore, learning for high-risk organizations is severely constrained when the events of interest (e.g., accidents or catastrophic failures) are statistically infrequent or perceived to be rare. Even more challenging is how these organizations try to prevent the occurrence of a catastrophe. A new way of gaining knowledge is needed.

Key safety principles for system safety (Wilf–Mirron et al., 2003):

1. Errors inevitably occur and usually derive from faulty system design, not from negligence.
2. Accident prevention should be an ongoing process based on open and full reporting.
3. Major accidents are only the "tip of the iceberg."

Military and commercial aviation, nuclear power, and petrochemical industries are the undisputed leaders for expanding their learning ability from investigating actual adverse events to studying close calls. Experts in these industries admit that safety is not a choice and that one singular disaster in any one organization will have a negative impact on all organizations within the entire industry. It is no wonder that catastrophic events, such as Three Mile Island, Chernobyl, Bhopal, and Tenerife, registered so dreadfully and infamously. In health care, the comparison between the surgical theater and the cockpit has been referenced so often that most people have looked to the aviation industry for lessons that can be directly imported into health care. Without understanding the organizational environment and the root of the problem in health care, lessons learned from other successful industries may not always work as a panacea.

In 1974 during a final approach for landing, TWA Flight 514 crashed into a mountain in Virginia. Six weeks before this crash, the crew of United Airlines at the exact location experienced a similar danger, and the danger was communicated to other pilots of the company. The TWA crash prompted the Federal Aviation Administration (FAA) to implement a national incident reporting system as a means to collect information and improve flight safety. In May 1975, the FAA formally established the Aviation Safety Reporting Program with provisions of anonymity and limited immunity to any individual who submitted an incident report. This program became operational in 1976. However, few reports were filed because the potential reporters distrusted the FAA that regulates the air industry and enforces aviation regulations. To counter this barrier and improve reporting, in August 1975 the FAA contracted NASA as a neutral third party to develop and operate the Aviation Safety Reporting System (ASRS). Funded by the FAA, a prototype of ASRS was introduced in 1976 and has been fully operational since May 1978 (National Academy of Public Administration, 1994).

The ASRS today is often used as a model for other safety reporting systems. More than 30,000 reports of near midair collisions, altitude and heading deviations, runway incursions, and so forth are submitted yearly by pilots, air traffic controllers, and other flight operators. Contents of the ASRS reports are studied by safety analysts after personal identifiers (reporter's name, license number, airline, flight number, aircraft make, and tail number of aircraft) are removed. Important safety information is rapidly disseminated to the airlines and private pilots to improve safety. Often the information is used in training and simulation, as well as in changing and improving operational procedures and policies.

For most aviators and flight safety researchers, the ASRS is a relatively useful system to capture safety data. However, the baseline for reporting has never been established. Therefore, no one knows how to interpret why reporting goes up or down during any given month. ASRS reports should not be used as the only indicator of safety because many factors, such as stories and news coverage of a recent air disaster, can influence risk perception and reporting of close calls (Mireles, 1996). The number of reported incidents is only a conservative measure of the true number of incidents that occur.

Anyone involved in flight operations cannot be certain what part of the flight is under computer surveillance. Consequently, any flight violation can be monitored and further investigated by the FAA. Self-reports of flight violation to the ASRS can provide limited protection and immunity from FAA prosecution, if the report is submitted and documented within 10 days.

The Veterans Affairs (VA) health care system adopted the ASRS for patient safety using virtually the identical reporting structure involving NASA. The Patient Safety Reporting System (PSRS) was set up in 2002 as an external reporting system for the VA. Only about 400 PSRS reports were recorded in 2005 and 10 safety bulletins were issued to the network of VA hospitals (Clancy, 2008). The effectiveness of the PSRS is still undetermined, and it will take many more years to evaluate the robustness and utility of this safety reporting system.

Beyond Safety Reporting

As the airline industry evolved into an organization and culture of safety, a systems approach to complex problems has become the ideal method to better understand how parts are integrated and how they may fail causing disastrous consequences. As a former military pilot and accident investigation team leader for the Israeli Air Force, I introduced some concepts of systems thinking into our standard investigation protocol. Within 5 years of implementing a systems thinking approach to accident investigation and prevention, the accident rate in the Israeli Air Force was reduced by approximately 50 percent in 5 years (Wilf-Miron et al., 2003).

The systems approach steps introduced to achieve the reduction in accident rate were:

1. Create a training school for accident investigation, loss prevention, and root cause analysis.
2. Rewrite existing policies and procedures to reflect the spirit of the gradual organizational culture shift toward safety.
3. Classify and code reported events into categories so statistical analysis could be performed, trends identified, and potential threats of an aviation accident identified.
4. Design, develop, and populate a software system using the classification and coding system described in step 3.
5. Encourage and reward proactive, preventive action, and minimize punitive consequences to individuals at the sharp end for design and system failures.
6. Continually educate personnel that human error is almost always a result of failure of management and the system, and be accepted as a standard way to gradually improve processes in order to enhance the quality of outcomes.

The prerequisite for these changes is having the organizational culture and support to make the changes, improve operations, and continually learn. Organizations want to improve and grow, but they usually lack the ability to learn and build experiences. Most will focus only on short-term solutions and fail to create the behavior that can be sustained over time. Based on my experience, the heart of continual improvement and organizational learning is communication, which encompasses more than data collection and analysis. Communication should be pervasive, rich, transparent, effective, and meaningful from the individual to the organization so that everyone in the system can share a role in learning and improving the system. The PSO provides an essential foundation for better communication in our health care system.

To achieve the level of communication that can vastly enhance our health care quality and patient safety, successful transition from our current disparate systems based on just reporting medical errors, near misses, "never" events, and so forth, to open communication among all individuals, groups, at all levels within the organization, I proposed the following key elements:

1. Create an entity independent of all the functions/silos/departments/institutions and be responsible only to the CEO of the entire system.
2. The purpose of all investigations would be for performance improvement and safety, not for punitive purposes.
3. All information gathered used for safety, quality, and safety improvement could not be used in litigation or in punitive measures.
4. All recommendations based on the outcomes of the research and investigations would be shared and learned or taught to all parties involved irrespective of their duties or functions directly connected to the case at hand.

The challenges currently faced in health care are the same as those faced in the Israeli Air Force or any high-risk organization. Everyone had their own culture or tried to understand and also conform to the status quo, "the way we do things here." Changes are considered disruptive to operations, and leaders, commanders, and managers did not want to change the way things were done. The only way to convince them to change was to demonstrate a different way that would produce an optimal outcome.

The annual flight safety award in the Israeli Air Force traditionally is given to the squadron that has the least number of events. After introducing the new safety system, it was discovered that the squadron reporting the most near misses also experienced the lowest rate of accidents. Reporting of near misses with the new system is inversely related to the actual incidents. The culture of near-miss reporting expanded the discussion and analysis of potentially dangerous situations in flight, as well as the institutional learning that created an immediate impact on performance and improvement in our safety goals.

Building the PSO as an Integrated Quality Management and Communication System

The evolution of the PSO structure began before the Patient Safety Act of 2005, with only a handful of groups studying the origin and impact of medical error as an indicator of quality and safety of the health care system. Several models of the PSO are expected to emerge among various competing vendors. Concurring with Carolyn Clancy, director of AHRQ (2008), I predict four popular PSO models would include (1) health care systems creating their component PSO in partnership with other hospital systems, (2) national medical specialty societies and professional groups that self-fund and operate their component PSOs, (3) independent medical consultant groups that will provide service for component PSOs to collect and study health information and improve health care quality and patient safety, and (4) a consortium of state PSOs connected to and forming the national PSO. The third model will provide a comprehensive and customized suite of patient safety work product tools and patient safety evaluation systems (PSES) to achieve the common format for PSOs.

The PSO Services Group (PSO 28) is comprised of diversified patient safety professionals who have designed innovative and modern technologies to provide services that meet the recommendations of the IOM studies *To Err is Human* (2000), *Crossing the Quality Chasm* (2001), and *Building a Better Delivery System* (2005).

Learning organizations are skilled at:

■ Systematic problem solving
■ Experimenting with new approaches
■ Learning from their own experiences and past history

- Learning from experiences and best practices of others
- Transforming knowledge quickly and efficiently throughout the organization to improve performance (Smith, 1995)

CRG Medical has built a healthcare information company, designed an adaptable system to scale in size from 25-bed critical access hospitals to a nationwide PSO system. This application alone has taken almost 4 years to build and integrate all the necessary parts of an integrated communication and learning system.

Rather than a simple network of component PSOs connecting health providers and the DHHS, I envision the creation of a multilayered organization of PSOs. One or more Super PSOs positioned at the state or regional level will oversee the operations and activities or network of PSOs within a defined geographical area. Some smaller states and territories may be combined into one Super PSO, while more populous states will set up more than one Super PSO. These Super PSOs serve as the final gatekeepers to ensure the quality and reliability of patient safety data, and they will comprise the elements of the Network of Patient Safety Databases to house important data and discoveries.

The Super PSO shown in Figure 12.1, the Maine PSO network, is the large, more expansive network of PSOs working directly with health providers (hospitals) to collect and process patient safety data. In some cases, the PSO may be a virtual entity with members from health provider organizations working collaboratively using the latest communication technology. The two levels of PSOs are defined as the PSO network. Depending on the number of PSOs and the size and complexity of the PSO network, a third and even a fourth level may be considered.

Information will flow upward and downward freely between the Super PSOs and the network of PSOs under the auspices and protection of federal statute provided in the Patient Safety Act. For the first time, lessons learned about a dangerous event in one hospital can be quickly communicated or shared with other hospitals to prevent harm and transform best practices to best processes for

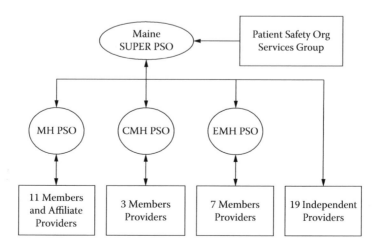

Figure 12.1   The Maine patient safety organization network.

safety. Hospitals can become true learning organizations. Awareness, education, and training would be required to encourage communicating actual adverse and near-miss events.

The organizational chart in Figure 12.1 shows the proposed PSO network that is being considered for the state of Maine with three defined network divisions involving some 40 hospitals: Maine Health PSO, Central Maine Health PSO, and Eastern Maine Health PSO.

In addition to setting this PSO network in Maine as the first state model for the nation, the PSO Services Group will recommend and assist in the creation of an independent PSO advisory committee or board that would include key players and stakeholders, including the Maine Medical Society, Maine Department of Health and Human Services, and reputable higher education institutions involved in health sciences. Ideally, the University of Maine would be the best candidate to collaborate in this endeavor. Other states might consider a university or health science center with an established medical school or health science curriculum to be involved with the planning and implementation of the PSO and related research activities.

The Final Rule of the Patient Safety and Quality Improvement Act of 2005 was published January 19, 2009. Anyone and any organization that intends to apply for and register as a PSO should demonstrate the following service capabilities:

1. Design a Web-based communication system for sending the "patient safety work product" to the component PSO of each hospital system.
2. Design a Web-based analytical system to aggregate the patient safety data that would serve as part of the Patient Safety Evaluation System.
3. Create an expert system to build and support institutional and organizational knowledge from gathered patient safety data and information, and to share this knowledge with member providers.
4. Create a set of policies, consistent and compatible with the Final Rule and the legal jurisdiction of each participating state and component PSO from each hospital system.
5. Partner with a health care compliant data warehouse to provide reliable and secure hosting and backup services.

The Patient Safety Organization Services Group and CRG Medical based in Houston are already leading the research and national effort to help organize and implement the patient safety organization. Those structures are positioned to become the engine for the entire PSO system and help transform hospitals into learning organizations with improved quality management and communication systems.

The center of this engine is the KBCore System for patient safety information communication, data aggregation, performance analysis, and best process knowledge feedback. Other analytical patient safety work products and components of the group include Peer Review, the C-Suite Patient Safety Decision Making Dashboards, and the customized Quality Care System (QCS) that will include Physician Quality Reporting Initiative (PQRI) for Category II quality data. Health providers can take advantage of subscribing to the supplemental patient safety platforms and services, such as the CMS HCAHPS Surveys, Web-based AHRQ Patient Safety Culture Surveys, Leadership Assessments and Diagnostics, Risk Assessment Profile Analysis, Baldrige Performance Excellence preparation consulting, and architectural support in patient safety design and construction of health care facilities. One added benefit of Patient Safety Services Group as a PSO provider is the research support provided by partner Community Medical Foundation for Patient Safety, a proven leader in patient safety and health care systems research. This network of services is growing fast to bring in new partnerships with other leaders in patient safety and health care quality.

Notes

To learn more about the Patient Safety and Quality Improvement Act of 2005, visit http://ww.pso.ahrq.gov/contact/contact/htm or contact the chapter author Douglas Dotan at dotan@swbell.net or visit http://www.psoservices.net.

References

Agency for Healthcare Research and Quality. The Patient Safety and Quality Improvement Act of 2005. http://www.ahrq.gov/qual/psoact.htm (accessed June 2008).

Clancy CM. New patient safety organizations lower roadblocks to medical error reporting. *Am J Medical Qual*, Jul/Aug 2008, 23(4), 318–321.

Dotan D. Communities of competence: A concept behind implementation of quality improvement and patient safety centers in health care. *Am Soc for Qual Health Care Division Newsletter*, Spring 2002, 10–11.

Dotan D. A systems approach to patient safety and the delivery of health care. *J Qual Health Care*, April/June 2004, 20–25.

Greenberg J and Baron RA. *Behavior in organizations: Understanding and managing the human side of work*. Prentice Hall, New Jersey, 2000, 601–602.

Institute of Medicine. *To Err is Human*. National Academies Press, Washington, DC, 2000.

Institute of Medicine. *Crossing the Quality Chasm: A New Health System for the 21st Century*. National Academies Press, Washington, DC, 2001.

Institute of Medicine. *Building a Better Delivery System: A New Engineering/Health Care Partnership*. National Academies Press, Washington, DC, 2005.

Mireles MC. Accidents in the news: A study of NASA Aviation Safety Reporting System for individual and organizational learning. University of Texas Health Science Center, School of Public Health, master's thesis, 2006, 7–9.

National Academy of Public Administration. A review of the Aviation Safety Reporting System: A report by a study team of the National Academy of Public Administration for the Federal Aviation Administration, 1994.

Smith EA. The challenge of the learning organization. *The Qual Observer*, 1995.

Wilf-Miron R, Lewenhoff I, Benyamini Z and Aviram A. From aviation to medicine: Applying concepts of aviation safety to risk management in ambulatory care. *Qual Saf Health Care*, 2003, 12, 35–39.

Chapter 13

Alternative Emergency Care Settings

James Lifton

Introduction

Hospital-based emergency departments accommodate over 119 million patient visits annually,[1] and physicians and other clinicians working there save countless lives. Emergency departments (EDs) have resources and services that are not available anywhere else. For people suffering from acute injury or illness, they are an indispensable part of the health care delivery system.

However, EDs are routinely called on to provide general medical services and care for patients that they are not intended to care for. The traditional ED may not be able to meet these patients' needs, including a medical home[2] for follow-up care. And, the space, time, and staff that nonurgent patients use may make it more difficult for those in need of emergency care to receive service. A recent study found that waiting times for heart attack patients have increased much more than for ED patients overall, and concluded that "overcrowding... might be worsening care for those with truly urgent conditions."[3] So, providing care outside of the ED for nonemergent patients has the potential to improve their care as well as the care given to more seriously ill patients remaining in the ED.

The threat of sanctions under the Emergency Medical Treatment and Active Labor Act of 1986 (EMTALA) makes it unlikely that patients will be turned away from an ED, no matter what their medical condition. As a consequence, patients without the ability to pay for services, and perhaps without the need for emergency care, are drawn to EDs. (It should be noted that the increase in ED visits, at least through 2004, was found to be due largely to nonpoor patients.[4] So, while there is a financial burden in caring for uninsured or underinsured patients in the ED, it has not increased in proportion to the insured ED population.)

Overcrowded EDs with long waiting times seem to be the rule rather than the exception. Overcrowding is often the consequence of conditions outside of the ED, especially the lack of inpatient beds. These conditions, as well as processes within the department, can and should be improved.[5] However, even an ED with optimal patient flow may have inadequate capacity.

Some hospitals have developed a fast-track component of the ED where, following triage, patients who don't need emergency care and resources are seen. This approach can reduce waiting times for nonemergent patients and can be a more economical way to deliver care than in the main ED. However, challenges such as providing follow-up care and collecting for services are not addressed by this approach.

While there is often no substitute for emergency care, four other settings have some features that could position them as complements, perhaps in some instances as alternatives, to hospital-based EDs. They include:

1. Freestanding emergency centers
2. Federally Qualified Health Centers
3. Urgent care centers
4. Convenient care clinics

Freestanding Emergency Centers

A freestanding emergency center is a facility that provides comprehensive emergency treatment services 24 hours per day on an outpatient basis. Such a facility is separate from, but affiliated with, a hospital and has a transfer arrangement to accommodate any emergency visits that result in inpatient admission. Freestanding emergency centers are regulated by state licensure laws, which typically require that they are equipped like a hospital ED and staffed by physicians. Because of the cost to build, equip, and operate, these facilities are expensive and have limited applicability as alternative emergency care settings.

The American Hospital Association reports that there are fewer than 200 freestanding emergency centers and there has been little growth in their number. Freestanding emergency centers have been developed most often to serve an area with limited hospital access. This may be a growing area where the hospital is looking to establish a presence. Some hospitals have expanded the services offered at the freestanding emergency center, including establishing a new (or replacement) hospital.

Federally Qualified Health Centers

Federally Qualified Health Centers (FQHC), including community health centers and other safety net providers, are intended to enhance the provision of primary health services in underserved urban and rural communities. FQHCs often receive grant funding through the Public Health Service, but may also qualify by subcontracting to a grantee or meeting certain other conditions.[6] Health centers, now called FQHCs, date back to 1962. There are now some 1,150 such centers, operating 6,000 sites, caring for over 16 million people.

FQHCs are reimbursed for their costs when treating a patient covered by Medicare or Medicaid. The cost of uninsured patients is covered by the federal grant, other grants, gifts, or income derived from caring for commercially-insured patients.

FQHCs offer a wide range of services and are designed to be a patient's medical home. Thus, FQHC patients have a source for follow-up care subsequent to an ED visit. These patients might also be able to avoid an emergency visit through preventive care or by seeing a FQHC physician or other provider instead of going to the ED. FQHCs are well positioned to impact ED utilization, in that their target patient population—the uninsured and Medicaid beneficiaries—typically rely on the ED for more of their ambulatory care than privately insured and Medicare beneficiaries.

A recent report on the potential for FQHCs to reduce inappropriate ED utilization[7] found that:

- At least one-third of all ED visits are avoidable and could have been treated appropriately in a primary care setting.
- The cost of these avoidable visits was $18 billion.
- FQHCs could save Medicaid approximately $4 billion annually by reducing avoidable ED visits.
- Patients served by health centers have fewer preventable ED visits than those in underserved areas without a health center.

Reducing avoidable ED visits requires a formal diversion program, characterized by a strong, defined relationship between a health center and hospital. Examples of approaches used by FQHCs as part of a formal diversion program include: developing a care coordination program for frequent users of ED services, renting space within a hospital to deliver primary care, implementing a nurse triage call line, and utilizing an electronic referral system to direct patients from the ED to the health center and then make follow-up appointments.

Challenges in establishing an effective ED diversion program through a FQHC include:

- FQHC hours of operation, which are typically weekdays and do not offer a ready alternative for patients coming to the ED at night or on weekends.
- Lack of start-up funding, including funding for additional providers, extended hours, and for a patient education program regarding appropriate use of the ED.
- Information technology linking the hospital and FQHC, and facilitating continuity of care.

Establishing a FQHC is time consuming and governance requirements for FQHCs dictate that they are independent of hospitals. So, while it is possible to establish a FQHC (or FQHC look-alike, which is not grant funded but is eligible for cost reimbursement), this is a practical alternative to the ED only where there is an existing health center.

Urgent Care Centers

Urgent care centers, sometimes called immediate care centers, are facilities that care for patients who have an injury or illness that requires immediate care, but is not serious enough to warrant an ED visit. Urgent care centers are typically staffed by a physician and provide walk-in, extended-hour access to care for acute illnesses and injuries that are either beyond the scope or availability of the typical primary care practice or retail clinic. Urgent care covers the majority of acute care services in a more cost effective and efficient way than the typical ED. There are over 8,000 urgent care centers;[9] most are hospital-owned or affiliated.

Urgent care centers can help to improve both access to care and proper utilization of health care resources. They provide patients with medical attention for a large number of acute conditions when primary physicians may be unavailable or unable to treat, and when an emergency room visit is not necessary.

Convenient Care Clinics

Convenient care clinics, also known as retail clinics, are small facilities located in high traffic retail settings such as drugstores and food stores. They offer non-emergency health care to people who would otherwise have to wait for an appointment with their physician, who have no primary care physician, or who might otherwise go to an ED for nonurgent care.

Convenient care clinics are typically open seven days a week and have evening hours. They are usually staffed by advanced practice nurses or physician assistants who offer care for common episodic ailments including colds, flu, rashes, and muscles strains or sprains. Convenient care clinics may also offer immunizations, physicals, and health screenings. The services provided by a convenient care clinic are often identified on a sign or brochure at the facility. Initially, these facilities required payment at the time of service, although some health plans are including them as covered providers.

The convenient care industry began in 2000 when the first convenient care clinics, operated by QuickMedx, were opened in Minneapolis-St. Paul.[10] There are approximately 1,200 convenient care clinics in operation in 32 states. Most are owned by for-profit companies, and hospitals and physicians view them as competitors. However, some hospitals and systems have developed affiliation agreements with convenient care clinics and have begun to include them in their continuum of care.

Challenges to Establishing Alternative Emergency Care Settings

Levels of care offered in alternative emergency care settings overlap with one another and with the ED, and can be confusing, as can the financial arrangements associated with each level and setting. A recent study from the Department of Health and Human Services, referenced in *Healthy People 2010*, found that the majority of adults lack health literacy, defined as the capacity to "obtain, process and understand basic health information and services needed to make appropriate health decisions." So any program involving an emergency care setting will require a patient education program.

Some alternative emergency care settings, especially urgent care centers and convenient care clinics, compete with physician office practices. Before a hospital, or other organization with physician stakeholders, gets involved in these settings, physicians' interests must be taken into consideration.

When patients receive care at multiple sites and from multiple providers, it becomes more difficult to coordinate that care and document it in the patient's health record. This increases the need for information technology that interfaces with multiple providers.

Notes and References

1. Pitts, S., Niska, R., et. al. National Hospital Ambulatory Medical Care Survey: 2006 Emergency Department Summary. National Health Statistics Report, No. 7. August 6, 2008.
2. For a description of the medical home, see Joint Principles of the Patient-Centered Medical Home. American Academy of Family Physicians, American Academy of Pediatrics, American College of Physicians, American Osteopathic Association. March 2007.
3. Wilper, A., Woolhandler, S., et. al. Waits to See an Emergency Department Physician: U.S. Trends and Predictors, 1997–2004. Health Affairs (web exclusive). January 15, 2008.
4. Weber, E. Showstack, J., et. al. Are the Uninsured Responsible for the Increase in Emergency Department Visits in the United States? Annals of Emergency Medicine. April 2008.
5. Emergency Department Crowding: High Impact Solutions. American College of Emergency Physicians. April 2008.
6. Federally Qualified Health Center Fact Sheet. Center for Medicare & Medicaid Services. April 2008.
7. Choudhry, L., Douglass, M., et al. The Impact of Community Health Centers & Community-Affiliated Health Plans on Emergency Department Use. Association for Community Affiliated Plans and National Association of Community Health Centers, Inc. April 2007.
8. Issue Brief. Health Center-Hospital Affiliation Opportunities under the Deficit Reduction Act. National Association of Community Health Centers. April 2007.
9. Urgent Care Association of America, www.ucaoa.org.
10. Convenient Care Association, www.ccaclinics.org.

Appendix: Case Study— Surviving and Thriving in Emergency Department Chaos

Community General Hospital was experiencing serious delays in delivering patient care in its emergency department (ED). Primary indicators of the problem were: (1) increased throughput times for both emergency and minor care patients, (2) increased numbers of registered patients leaving the ED without having received treatment, (3) lack of sufficient space for patients (and the people who brought them) to wait until they are treated and released, (4) comments of frustration to hospital administrators by ED physicians and staff, and (5) a noticeable increase in negative comments on patient-satisfaction questionnaires returned by patients who had recently utilized the ED facilities. Minor tinkering with the standard operational procedures at that time gave only minor relief, and the problem persisted and grew worse annually.

Initial assessments indicated that the bottleneck primarily was due to rapidly increasing numbers of patients annually and lack of sufficient space to provide care to the increased number of patients presenting to the ED. Sufficient numbers of ED physicians, registered nurses, and all other necessary ancillary and support staff were available but could not attend to the patients in an efficient manner. The long-term solution to the bludgeoning annual growth rate was construction of a new ED facility. Strategic long-range planning for major capital projects had been completed and a new facility for the ED had been approved for completion, estimated to be in 5 years. Therefore, this ED needed a radical solution to get it through its crisis until the completion of the new facility.

An in-depth review of the ED situation by senior management, key staff, emergency physicians, and specially selected other personnel who were selected for their problem-solving abilities and their positive attitudes revealed several significant facts that were important in understanding the ED service problems. In spite of the approximately 10 percent annual growth over the past several years, projections for the next 5 years were for a continuing growth of 10 percent to 15 percent in ED volume per year. Review of diagnosis data revealed that 60 percent to 65 percent of patients in the ED were nonacute, in part due to insufficient primary care physicians in the community, few accessible minor medical care facilities, and other typical reasons. The hospital space comprising the ED was not designed to handle the current, much less the projected, volumes. Lower acuity patients comprised about 36,000 of the 71,000 visits per year, and the overwhelming volume of complaints about ED services came from these patients who experienced excessive waits, as much as 5 to 6 hours for some patients.

Purpose of Case Study

The purpose of this case study is to provide a rubric to hospital administrators seeking to provide a short-term solution to this and similar problems while strategically developing a long-range solution. Neither new construction nor immediate renovation was desirable without proper long-range strategic planning, but it was obvious that the short-term solution could only be accomplished through major revisions of triage, admission, and patient treatment workflow processes and procedures. In other words, the hospital's ED for the next 5 years had to do more, utilizing the same basic physical structure and square footage that had been identified earlier as the major limitation factor.

Definitions of Significant Terms

For purposes of understanding the important terminology used in this case study, the following terms are defined:

emergency department—An emergency department (commonly referred to as an *emergency room* by many patients) is a semiautonomous division of a typical hospital that is staffed 24 hours per day, 7 days per week, including holidays. Originally designed to primarily handle only emergency situations, it now is viewed by many in the general public as a place to be seen by a doctor within just a few hours, rather than have to wait days or weeks to get an appointment with a general practitioner or a specialist. For people without a family doctor, an emergency department often is their primary or only source of medical assistance. For those without insurance or who use public health facilities during regular hours, emergency departments fill the gap after hours.

one-track ED model—This term is used in reference to the traditional emergency department process for seeing patients who come for medical treatment. Emergency cases are seen on a priority basis, but nonemergency cases can also be seen as medical assistance becomes available. Both emergency and nonemergency patients, along with their friends and families, congregate in the same waiting room. Nonemergency patients typically have to wait to be called back to an available room for treatment, while true emergency patients are taken to a treatment room immediately. Registration normally is done at a desk while the patient waits in a waiting room to be called for treatment. Physicians who treat emergency patients also treat non-emergency patients.

two-track ED model—This term is used to describe an emergency department that is divided into two very distinct and separate treatment areas: one to treat emergency cases and one to treat nonemergency cases. A quick triage is performed upon patient entry through a single portal; this determines whether the patient is directed to the emergency care area or the nonemergency area. Rooms, physicians, and staff are assigned only to one (minor care or emergency/urgent) track, under normal circumstances.

patient-focused care—The basic rationale for patient-focused care is that as many services as economically feasible are brought to the patient, rather than have the patient directed to separate desks and areas within the ED or other departments for registration, treatment, ancillary services, certain x-ray and laboratory services, discharge, and so forth.

cross-trained staff—In essence, cross-training of staff provides a wider diversity of skills to a team of caregivers. This allows the staff to prevent delays by providing multiple services in a timely manner. While recognizing that not all staff members have the capability to perform all of the duties and responsibilities of specialized coworkers, this concept requires the training of ED staff members to do as many functions as they can do that normally are performed by other coworkers who have different job titles and responsibilities. For example, a registered nurse (RN) may be cross-trained to perform respiratory therapist procedures as well as some lab functions; an ED tech may perform the role of a phlebotomist as well as transport patients to the radiology department for an x-ray procedure; and unit secretaries can be cross-trained to perform some business office functions for other staff members. Cross-trained staff speed the delivery of necessary services to the patients, because there is no wait for specialized personnel to arrive from another part of the ED, hospital, or from being on call to the ED. It must be noted, however, that there are a few situations in which licensure requirements prevent a person from performing certain functions, even when the unlicensed person can perform the desired tasks adequately. State boards for licensure rules and regulations should be reviewed and questioned prior to finalizing new job descriptions addressing cross-training issues.

emergency patients—This term specifically refers to those patients in ED facilities who face life-threatening medical problems, severe pain, or further medical harm if not seen immediately by a skilled physician. Since assignment to an emergency track is based upon the availability of treatment rooms and physicians, as well as by initial triage assessment, patients who might otherwise be among the more severe of the nonemergency cases may be assigned to the emergency track in order to utilize both tracks efficaciously.

The true emergency patients are also referred to as *critical care patients* and *acute care patients.*

minor care patients—These are patients whose symptoms/health complaints are not among the more severe. Occasionally, the very least severe of these patients may have to wait longer than usual to be treated, even in the minor care facility. These patients are also referred to as *nonacute patients, non-emergency patients,* and *noncritical patients.*

Background of the Problem

Community General Hospital (CGH) is located in a small city of 85,000 people, surrounded by a larger and mainly rural service area. CGH's primary service area contains a population of approximately 200,000 people, with a combined primary and secondary market of 675,000 within a 55-mile radius. With a total of more than 250 physicians on its staff, CGH offers a wide range of programs and services. It provides a continuum of care that addresses nearly the full spectrum of health care needs of people within its primary and secondary markets.

CGH is a 450-bed nonprofit, tertiary medical center, designated as a level 2 trauma center. The ED is staffed by an independent physician group, consisting of 20 members who contract their services to the hospital.

As the enormity of the ED's problem surfaced initially, the ED reported a volume of almost 71,000 patient visits each year; and each year for the preceding several years the volume had increased by approximately 10 percent per year. With this continuing growth, the throughput times and other negative indicators had increased concurrently. Along the way, CGH had made varying attempts to rectify the problem with minor changes, which resulted in minor improvements but had not alleviated the problem significantly. Thus, over the ensuing years the continually increasing throughput times and their consequences had now resulted in unacceptable results.

CGH had always treated all patients presenting to the ED regardless of their ability to pay or their acuity level. Those with acute life-threatening situations have always been given first priority to be seen by the medical staff. That group, of course, was and is the rationale for the existence of emergency departments. Technically, all other patients are generally categorized as nonemergency. While that may be true technically, in reality, second priority is given to those patients with acute but not life-threatening symptoms. Finally, persons not meeting the criteria for either of the first two groups comprise the minor care patients. This group frequently experiences long waits to receive medical attention due to priority being given to the true emergencies and to the more acute/urgent cases.

Today, more than ever, many nonemergency patients who previously would have been seen primarily by family practice physicians or specialists during regular office hours are now often being seen primarily by ER doctors. This last group has continued to grow at a faster rate than any of the other groups or categories, and it is this group that has most contributed to the overflows in many emergency departments across America.

A formalized process for soliciting patient evaluations of Community General's services, procedures, and other factors had been in effect for many years. Questionnaires were mailed to the home within 2 weeks of a patient's discharge from the ED. Patients were asked to rate many specified components with an assigned rating scale and also asked to write individual comments as they chose. The returned questionnaires were scanned and tabulated to discern trends of problems as well as areas of strength within a period of just a few weeks. From observation of the tabulated responses, negative comments regarding the ED were growing rapidly. Furthermore, the ED personnel (both the physicians and the staff) also were aware of patient concerns and were themselves becoming quite frustrated with their inability to provide their usual level of care within appropriate time frames and with acceptable patient satisfaction responses.

Methods and Procedures

Senior hospital administration, eschewing a quick fix, was determined to find the best solutions within the limited time and monies available for renovation. As was its normal procedure when faced with problems of such magnitude, administration's decision was to secure the assistance of outside consultants with expertise in such matters. The consultants were challenged with the tasks of redesigning workflow processes and standard operating procedures within the existing ED space that would significantly: (1) improve the velocity (throughput times), (2) improve patient satisfaction scores, and (3) decrease the numbers of patients leaving the ED without receiving treatment.

At this point the consultants requested CGH supply them with copious amounts of specified documents, including architectural plans, time and motion studies, manuals of standard operating procedures associated with the ED and all ancillary and associated departments and groups, job descriptions, and so forth. After receiving these, the consultants requested other such materials over the next few weeks that they deemed significant to their task.

Meanwhile, at CGH, intradepartmental focus groups were established to identify inefficiencies in workflow processes and to redesign those processes within the ED as well as in other pertinent clinical and support departments. Work groups from the following departments or units were created to study existing workflow processes that affected the efficiency of work within the ED and also to suggest solutions on ways to positively impact efficiency within their own work unit/department to better serve the ED and its patients: ED physicians, ED nurses, ED staff (other than physicians and nurses), radiology, respiratory therapy, registration/admission, clinical information systems, ED host, radiology, case mix analysis, quality assurance, laboratory, and discharge. In addition to these focus groups, other focus groups (human resources, employee health, direct admit, etc.) consisting only of specific departmental staff were set up for the review of activities occurring in the ED that were not essential to the care of ED patients.

After an in-depth review and evaluation of the work of the focus groups; the background data that the hospital provided; and concerns of staff, physicians, and administration, the consultants presented their findings, conclusions, and recommendations. In their presentation to the hospital, they first identified areas of major strengths and weaknesses of the ED. Areas of weakness provided opportunities for improvement and became the focus for the recommended redesign of the ED. The weaknesses identified were: (1) throughput times were increasing to a level that was not longer acceptable to the patients be served by this ED; (2) patient satisfaction had declined to an unacceptable level; (3) staff satisfaction had declined in direct proportion to the declining patient satisfaction; (4) ED rooms were not being properly utilized as a result of patient delays and increasing length of stay in the ED; ED physical space, which was originally built in the early 1960s for an annual volume of 35,000 (and had only minor updates through the years), was no longer adequate for the present and projected future volumes.

Once the opportunities for improvement were clearly identified, the challenges that lay ahead for this ED also became quite clear. The administration quickly realized that the solutions would require committed leadership as well as an intradepartmental commitment for organizational change to be able to create new ways of conducting work in the ED. It was decided to deploy the same intradepartmental focus groups used during the initial assessment and evaluation of the problem phase to continue as the redesign teams. Their charge was to review the present way work was performed, evaluate workflow, identify inefficiencies, and redesign work flow to be significantly more efficient.

The first initiatives to be studied in detail for redesign were the various stages of patient flow: (1) triage; (2) registration; (3) assessment; (4) diagnosis and treatment; and (5) disposition. Background data, workflow studies, and time studies were conducted for each of the stages of patient flow. Examination of the existing processes reflected unnecessarily long and fragmented approaches to patient care with the triage, registration, and assessment stages. These three components were found to be the areas with the greatest negative effects upon throughput times. These were followed in decreasingly negative effects by the diagnosis and treatment stage and last by the disposition stage. Also discovered in this review, although not surprising to anyone, was that emergency patients were handled in the most efficient manner in all phases. Conversely, the lowest acuity patients were handled in the least efficient manner in all phases investigated.

In the traditional departmental one-track model previously used by CGH's emergency department, an incoming patient frequently had to travel between and among departments or "desks." A patient was expected to go to one desk for triage, another for registration; wait in a waiting room; then wait in an examining room; wait for a physician visit and to order tests; wait for the tests to be done; wait for the phlebotomist to come from the laboratory; wait for respiratory therapy, EKG, radiology, and so forth; wait to be transported to other departments for treatment such as x-ray; wait again in examining rooms; wait for results of tests and procedures; wait again for the physician and nurse to determine course of treatment and disposition; and finally wait some more to be discharged.

After extensive review of these workflow processes and their effects upon efficiency, patient satisfaction, and throughput times, the following recommendations were submitted and approved for implementation:

1. Use a rapid (implement all approved changes in 6 months) redesign approach.
2. Develop a treatment track for minor care patients separate from the emergency track, thus creating a two-track ED model.
3. Improve efficiency and reallocate staff procedures and responsibilities for "nonemergency" services.
4. Improve the throughput times for all ED patients by streamlining procedures among departments serving all ED patients.
5. Evaluate all redesign efforts and recommendations using the patient-focused principles listed next:
   a. All services will be taken to the patient, except when cost was prohibitive.
   b. All services will be provided by cross-trained ED personnel, unless prohibited by licensure.
   c. No services will be delivered in a defined sequence, unless required by standard operational procedure, in order to prevent delays in providing care.
   d. Only highly specialized functions will remain in centralized departments.
   e. The numbers of staff members interacting with the patient will be fewer—but more efficient—as a result of cross-training.

The patient-focused model uses a mini-triage system that was developed to provide an initial clinical screen in which a RN sorts and assigns incoming patients to the appropriate treatment area (minor care or emergency track) with no delays or waits at the time of entry to the ED. Then, following mini-triage, a patient is assigned to a treatment room in the minor care or emergency track depending upon severity of illness and is not sent to a waiting room, unless all treatment rooms are full.

In the redesigned patient-focused two-track model there now are two distinct and separate patient areas: a minor care track and an emergency track. Emergency department personnel designed workflow charts that showed patient flow for each of the following five stages: triage, registration, assessment, diagnosis and treatment, and disposition.

Prior to the redesign of the ED, the registration and assessment stages also resulted in significant patient delays. Using the principles of a patient-focused model, the registration process was changed from the traditional registration desk model to a bedside registration model in which patient registration occurred in the treatment room. Although there is a mini-assessment by a RN upon patient entry to the ED, there is an in-depth assessment by another RN after the patient is assigned to a treatment room. For each track, the RNs receiving and assessing the patients in the treatment room are empowered through the use of physician-approved protocols to order appropriate diagnostic studies/tests. With this standard operational procedure, patients are ready for medical diagnosis and treatment by a physician as early in the process as possible. Furthermore, this technique better utilizes the expertise and time of both RNs and ED physicians, and nurse practitioners.

The physical structure of the ED was redesigned to accommodate the patient-focused two-track delivery system. First, due to the increasing numbers of lower acuity patients being treated in the ED, eight additional minor care treatment rooms were added by utilizing space previously used as a large waiting room. Second, a new waiting area for the families of minor care patients was built adjoining, but completely separate from, the urgent/emergency patient family waiting area.

Having completely separate facilities for the patients and families of the more acute and the less acute cases was purposely designed to prevent the most frequent waiting room problem occurring under the one-track delivery system. Patients, families, and friends of the less acute patients often had been angered and had questioned why some patients were treated and released faster than other patients. Their impression too often was that the ED policy should be first come, first served without exception, other than life-threatening emergencies.

Under the new two-track system, the emergency patients and their families are separated at mini-triage from the lower acuity patients and their families, and are sent to completely separate treatment areas for diagnosis and treatment. Consequently, after mini-triage, each group is associated only with its cohort group—either higher acuity or lower acuity. These two groups stay separated throughout treatment and then are discharged through separate exits.

Next, redesign of the workflow of the diagnosis and treatment phase was undertaken by the appropriate focus groups. The major redesign effort for this phase was the need for an overall improvement in the interfacing with ancillary departments (e.g., respiratory therapy, lab, and radiology). Both consultants and focus groups were guided by the principles that services would be taken to the patient except when costs prohibited it and that care would not be rigidly sequenced. Thus, certain functions should be flexibly sequenced to allow full usage of all phases and, thus, would speed the overall process. Luckily, it was determined to be unnecessary to change the physical location of radiology, since procedure rooms that supported the ED were next door to the ED and the turnaround time for radiology procedures were typically good.

Regarding radiology, however, it was noted that the transport time for this short distance was excessive due to the wait for transport personnel after the orders were placed for x-rays. Similar opportunities for improvements were also noted in the timeliness of lab specimen collecting, lab results reporting, EKG results, and respiratory therapy turnaround times. Consequently, it was determined to be necessary to develop metric standards for specimen collecting, delivery of specimens by the ED, testing and analysis, and results reporting to the ED by ancillary departments.

Disposition and discharge was the next stage identified for redesign. In the former system, disposition/discharge primarily had been providing instructions to the patient (or family) on how to care for the patient after discharge from the ED. Prior to redesign there was no attempt to collect payment for services rendered, set up a payment plan, or gather all the information needed for future billing purposes. Once treatment was completed, patients were simply discharged and transported out of the facility. The disposition/discharge stage was redesigned to include payment collection functions after treatment was completed. The patient was escorted from the ED treatment area to the ED business office area located within the ED where there was an attempt to receive payment or set up a payment plan and collect all information needed for billing of the unpaid balance.

The final step in the redesign was the thorough review of the care and services being delivered by ED staff. Emphasis was placed upon identifying those elements that could just as easily be performed by other departments of the hospital. Identified functions, several of which are listed next, were eventually reassigned to other departments or areas:

1. The *direct admit function* of the ED was reassigned to the outpatient admission area. This freed ED employees to do more ED-specific work. Previously, obstetrics patients and other such patients who were being admitted to the hospital from their admitting physician first flowed through the ED. A rapid admit process was designed in which the admitting physician contacts the admissions office/bed control where a bed is assigned and the admission paper work started. Now these patients no longer flow through ED. Instead, as the patient arrives at the Direct Admit Area, the paperwork is completed and the patient is taken directly to a regular hospital room. If patients are "stretcher-only" patients, they are sent directly to an assigned room and the registration is completed at the bedside. In addition, *obstetrics admits* now can be taken directly to labor and delivery and be formally admitted by the labor and delivery staff at the bedside. These changes eliminated the need for those patients to flow through the emergency department and disrupt the necessary work of the ED.

2. *Employee health* was another function that previously was a responsibility of the ED but now has been reassigned elsewhere. An employee health division was organized within the human resources (personnel) department, and a dedicated staff was assigned to perform the necessary personnel health functions such as TB (tuberculosis) tests, immunizations, communicable disease tracking and reporting, and other appropriate services previously handled by the ED. Prior to the reassignment, 10 to 15 hospital employees were seen on a daily basis for such services as "hallway consults," treatment for various aches and pains, and other time-wasting and staff-wasting functions of the ED. Furthermore, over 3,000 required TB skin tests were

performed and read for hospital employees on an annual basis in the ED. Note that none of these activities/visits were counted in the official numbers of patients seen by the ED.

Results and Conclusions

Although patient volume has continued to increase annually, the following results were achieved:

1. The overall throughput time for both emergency track and minor track patients was significantly reduced (actual results: 130 minutes for emergency/ urgent patients and 80 minutes for minor care track patients).
2. For both tracks, patient satisfaction increased to a level of "excellent."
3. Through the use of cross-training, the numbers of ER staff necessary to provide patient care for each patient were reduced.
4. Registration at the bedside in the treatment rooms was implemented successfully using wireless technology.
5. Patients leaving the ER without treatment were dramatically reduced (reduced by 70 percent).

As a result of closely monitoring patient satisfaction scores and patient comments after initiation of the changes discussed throughout this case study, it became obvious that at least one additional change needed to be made. Patients reported that they wanted to see a physician as early in the treatment process as possible. Consequently, the physicians and administrators agreed upon the goal that every patient would be seen by a physician in the treatment room within 15 minutes of arrival. Although patient satisfaction scores were already showing improvement, this change led to an even greater improvement in patient satisfaction.

Conclusions and Recommendations

The redesign of CGH's ED from a one-track to a two-track patient-focused model has continued to be a very successful endeavor. With the passage of each year the numbers of patients entering the ED continued to increase, thus putting more of a burden on the current facilities and ED staff. It must be pointed out, however, that the solutions reported here were always viewed as temporary solutions used to buy time. The long-term solution (a completely new ED facility) has now been realized, complete with lessons learned from the redesign project described in this case study being incorporated as a template and guiding principles of design for the new facility.

Continued commitment to improving quality services/improving efficiencies, decreasing throughput times, and increasing patient and staff satisfaction is an ongoing organizational commitment that requires ongoing assessment and evaluation for continuing improvement opportunities.

Changes and models discussed herein should have strong applicability for EDs at all hospitals. The solutions utilized at Community General Hospital were extremely useful in solving ED problems and should also be extremely useful to other types of medical facilities. Such changes should save the facility money on a long-term basis, but they certainly allow the facility to operate more efficiently and effectively on a daily basis.

Selected Bibliography

Periodicals

Bazarian, J.J., Schneider, S.M., Newman, V.J., and Chodosh, J. 1996. Do admitted patients held in the emergency department impact the throughput of treat-and-release patients? *Academic Emergency Medicine* 3 (December): 1113–1118.

Beed, J., and Howard, G. 1996. Re-engineering: Managing radical change. *Leadership in Health Services* 5 (March–April): 29–32, 36.

Benson, R., and Harp, N. 1994. Using thinking to extend continuous quality improvement. *Quality Letter of Healthcare Leadership* 6 (July–August): 17–24.

Boost Satisfaction: Combine ED, urgent care. 1997. *Patient-Focused Care* 5 (September): 99–102.

Coogan, N. 1996. A look at our new emergency department, New England Medical Center, Boston, Mass. *Journal of Emergency Nursing* 22 (April): 38A–41A.

Cooke, J., and Finneran, K. 1994. A clearing in the crowd: Innovations in emergency services. *Paper Service, United Hospital Fund of New York* (January): 1–43.

Covington, C., Erwin, T., and Sellers, F. 1992. Implementation of a nurse practitioner-staffed fast track. *Journal of Emergency Nursing* 18 (April): 124–131.

Deciding to expand? Run the numbers. 1998. *Patient-Focused Care and Satisfaction* 6 (August): 93–94.

ED redesign puts all patients on fast track. 1997. *Patient-Focused Care* 5 (August): 87–90.

Fernandes, C.M., Wuerz, R., Clark, S., and Djurdjev, O. 1999. How reliable is emergency department triage? *Annals of Emergency Medicine* 34 (August): 141–147.

Goldman, D.A., Saul, S.A., Parsons, S., Mansoor, C., Abbott, A., Damian, F., Young, G.J., Homer, C., and Caputo, G.L. 1993. Hospital-based continuous quality improvement: A realistic appraisal. *Clinical Performance in Quality Health Care* 1 (April–June): 69–80.

Gordon, J.A. 1999. The hospital emergency department as a social welfare institution. *Annals of Emergency Medicine* 33 (March): 321–325.

Gourlay, R. 1998. Re-engineering. *International Journal of Health Care Quality Assurance Incorporating Leadership in Health Services* 11 (November 3): 76.

Harrell, A. 1994. Building a patient record system: New information technologies will support development of patient-focused care. *Health Progress* 75 (April): 51–54.

Holahan, J., and Kim, J. 2000. Why does the number of uninsured Americans continue to grow? *Health Affairs* 19 (July-August): 188–196.

Jackson, G., and Andrew, J. 1996. Using a multidisciplinary CQI approach to reduce ER-to-floor admission time. *Journal of Healthcare Quality* 18 (May–June): 18–21.

Jaffe, D.T., and Scott, C. 1997. The human side of re-engineering. *Medicare Forum Journal* 40 (September–October): 14–21.

Karpiel, M.S. 1993. New service lines for hospital emergency departments. *Healthcare Financial Management* 47 (November): 40–44.

Lavary, R.R. 1997. Re-engineering hospital emergency rooms: An information system approach. *International Journal of Health Care Quality Assurance Incorporating Leadership in Health Services* 10 (4–5): 179–191.

Mezza, I. 1992. Triage: Setting priorities for health care. *Nursing Forum* 27 (April–June): 15–19.

Mowen, J.C., Licata, J.W., and McPhail, J. 1993. Waiting in the emergency room: How to improve patient satisfaction. *Journal of Health Care Marketing* 13 (Summer): 26–33.

O'Donnell, D. 1999. What works. Automated ER triage process saves money, speeds patient care. *Health Management Technology* 20 (June): 44–45.

Pardee, D.A. 1992. Decreasing the wait for emergency department patients: An expanded triage nurse role. *Journal of Emergency Nursing* 18 (August): 311–315.

Patrick, M., and Alba, T. 1994. Health care benchmarking: A team approach. *Quality Management of Health Care* 2 (Winter): 38–47.

Peterson, L.A., Burstin, H.R., O'Neil, A.C., Orav, E.J., and Brennan, T.A. 1998. Nonurgent emergency department visits: The effects of having a regular doctor. *Medical Care* 36 (August): 1249–1255.

Pierce, B., and Egging, D. 1994. Case studies in work redesign: "Do it yourself" redesign. *Journal of Emergency Nursing* 20 (October): 40A–42A.

Redesign triage areas for optimum efficiency. 1996. *ED Management: The Monthly Update on Emergency Department Management* 8 (June): 67–69.

Rizos, J., Anglin, P., Grava-Gubins, I., and Lazar, C. 1990. Walk-in clinics: Implications for family practice. *Canadian Medical Association Journal* 143 (October 15): 740–745.

Sainsbury, S.J. 1990. Emergency patients who leave without being seen: Are urgently ill or injured patients leaving without care? *Military Medicine* 155 (October): 460–464.

Sandrick, K. 1999. Moving patients through: Three top-performing emergency departments demonstrate how it's done. *Strategic Healthcare Excellence* 12 (July): 1–7.

Schaming, J.S., and Gulati, A. 1998. Health care quality improvement in the emergency department: A reengineering approach. *Top Health Information Management* 18 (May): 70–80.

Schneider, K.C. 1990. Medical review and the newly revised emergency care obligations of Medicare hospitals. *Quality Assurance and Utilization Review* 5 (August): 74–79.

Shumacher, W. 1999. Methods for improving emergency department operational process. *Health Care Strategic Management* 17 (February): 13–15.

Simon, H.K., Nordenberg, D.F., and Wright, J.A. 1997. Changes in academic emergency departments in response to market driven health care reform. *Academic Medicine* 72 (May): 44.

Sturmann, K.M., Ehrenberg, K., and Salzberg, M.R. 1990. Physician assistants in emergency medicine. *Annals of Emergency Medicine* 19 (March): 304–308.

Switching to bedside registration increases patient satisfaction. 1997. *ED Management* 9 (March): 25–30.

Travers, D. 1999. The triage: How long does it take? How long should it take? *Journal of Emergency Nursing* 25 (June): 238–240.

Trudeau, S., and Ladue, M. 1996. Wireless bedside registration in the ED. *Journal of Emergency Nursing* 22 (February): 57–60.

Vestal, K.W. 1983. Promoting excellence in the emergency department. *Journal of Emergency Nursing* 9 (September-October): 290–293.

Whipple T.W., and Edick, V.L. 1993. Continuous quality improvement of emergency services. *Journal of Health Care Marketing* 13 (Winter): 26–30.

Wright, S.W., Erwin, T.L., Blanton, D.M., and Covington, C.M. 1992. Fast track in the emergency department: A one-year experience with nurse practitioners. *Journal of Emergency Medicine* 10 (May–June): 367–373.

Books and Pamphlets

Matson, T.A. (editor). *The Hospital Emergency Department: A Guide to Operational Excellence.* American Hospital Publishing, Chicago, 1992.

Schloss, J. (editor). *Redefining the Emergency Department: Five Strategies for Reducing Unnecessary Visits.* The Advisory Board Co., Washington, DC, 1993.

Index

process simulation modeling, 11
real-time flow, 1–2
simulation modeling, 8–10
Six Sigma methodology, 5–7
statistical forecasting, 5
variation, 8
workload communication, 2
Emotional ties, 18, 198
Employee health, 217–218
EMTALA, *see* Emergency Medical Treatment
and Active Labor Act (EMTALA)
Engineered nurse staffing requirements
acuity systems, 184–186
arrival of patients, 184
developing requirements, 188–190
fundamentals, 190
predetermined treatment profiles, 189–190
ratio purpose, 183–184
service times, 186–187
time factors, 187–188
treatment profiles, 187
work sampling, 190
zero-based staffing approach, 189
Engineers, working with, 87–88
"Entourage" accompanying patients, 142
Environmental Adaptation Model, 333, *see
also* Complex adaptive systems
thinking
Environment of care, 69
Equity, 15, 193
Ergonomic factors, 188
Erlang studies, 117
Error of averages, 121
Errors, medical, 67, 191
Everything You Need To Know, 11
Excel software
analytic queuing models and DES, 117
congestion problem, 62
forecasting, 166
performance evaluation, 61
queuing model, 59–60
Experiments
simulation model planning, 86–87, 101–103
small scale, 46–47

F

FAA, *see* Federal Aviation Administration
(FAA)
Face-to-face meetings, 104
Falvo, Tom, 1–11, 244
Fast track processes, 56, 59, 204
Federal Aviation Administration (FAA), 195

Federally Qualified Health Centers (FQHC),
204–206
Feied, Smith and, studies, 81
Ferguson, Ginger, 245
Filming processes, 18
Final rule of the Patient Safety and Quality
Improvement Act (2005), 200
Fitzpatrick, Joyce, 107
Florida Sterling Quality Award, 33
Flowcharts, 16, 17, 21, *see also* Workflow
analysis and diagramming
Floyd Regional Medical Center, 42–43
Ford studies, 33
Forecasting
annual visits, 155–156
budgeting, 156–159
daily visits, 159–160
fundamentals, 154
hourly visits, 160–164
managing, 154
monthly visits, 156–159
physical capacity needs, 155–156
producing, 154
scheduling, 159–164
staffing, 156–160
using prediction intervals, 164
Fourier regression, 160–162
Freestanding emergency centers, 204
Front end, 1–11
Frontline staff members
collaboration, 23
observation affect on, 17–18
"seeing" processes, 15
workflow analysis, 16
Full/Busy Probability, 143
Future directions, 105
"Future state" diagrams, 16–17
Future steps, 52

G

Gap analysis, 144
George studies, 74
Giuliani, Lou, 5, 26
Goals
driving elements, Lean Six Sigma
methodologies, 41
ED triage, 1–2
"Going Lean In Health Care," 8
Goldman studies, 136
Good, Marion, 226
Good to Great, 40, 43
Goodwin, Debbie, 36

Roles
  nursing, 68–70
  senior leaders, 38–39
Roper, Nancy, 107
Rostering, 5, *see also* Scheduling
Routine activities, 186, 189
Rowe studies, 136
Roy, Callista, 107

S

Safety, *see also* Patient safety organizations
      (PSO)
  health care, 193
  processes quality, 15
Satisfaction reports, 84
Savings, 48–49, *see also* Costs
Scheduling, *see also* Self-scheduling approach
  completion stage, 173
  ESI case mix data impact, 5
  regression analysis, 159–164
  simulation modeling engineers, 87
SCHIP, *see* State Children's Health Insurance
      Program (SCHIP)
Schoenhofer, Savina, 106
Scope
  creep, electronic documents, 22
  lessons learned, 104
  simulation model planning, 86–87
Scoping, model, 83, 87
Sealed bid auction, 172, *see also* Auction
      approach
Sears, Doug, 23
Seasonality, 126, 130
Secondary peaks, 165
"Secrets of Great Healthcare Organizations,"
      39
"Seeing" processes, 15
Self-scheduling approach, *see also*
      Scheduling
  fundamentals, 170–171
  time demand, 178
  York Hospital case study, 174, 176
Senior leaders, 38–40
September 11, 2001, *x*
Sequences, observation, 19
Series processing, 36
Serious play
  process simulation, 119
  prototypes, 133
  service capacity, physiology, 128–130
  system balance, 131
Servers, 58

Service capacity, physiology, *see also* Capacity
  analytic queuing models, 117–118
  breaking points, 131
  capacity, 111–113
  confidence intervals, 114–115
  critical common resources, 130
  demand and capacity matching, 123–128
  demand patterns, 114–115
  discrete event simulation, 117–118
  dynamic capacity matching, 128–130
  dynamic resource allocation, 126–127
  fundamentals, 109–111, 124, 132
  granularity, 124–126
  HODDOW WOMSOY, 126–128
  interdependencies, 121–122
  patterns, 113–115
  physiology, 132
  predictive analytics, 122–123
  queuing theory and simulation, 116–117
  serious play, 128–130
  system balance, 128–132
  time, effect on processes, 122
  time stamps, 127–128
  "up-down-up" impacts, 123
  variability, 111–113, 116–121
  what-ifs, 122–123
Service rates, 59, 62
Service times, 186–187, *see also* Waiting and
      waiting times
Shiver, John M. (Jay), *vii–x*, 239
Shoot from the hip category, 44–45
Silos, 19
Simple regression analysis, 45
Simulation modeling
  barriers, 75
  capacity to serve, 9
  complexity, 10
  fundamentals, 8
  interconnectedness, 9
  interdependency, 9
  model run, 104
  Nightingale's approach, 70
  patient differences, 10–11
  variation, 8
Simulation modeling, planning
  animation, 99, 100
  approach, 78–79
  architectural data, 83–85
  case study, 88–101
  clinical data, 83–85
  complex adaptive systems thinking, 70–73
  data, 83–85
  database, 97–98

About the Editors

John M. (Jay) Shiver serves as an assistant professor in the Department of Health Administration and Policy at George Mason University, Fairfax, Virginia, where he teaches in the graduate and undergraduate programs. He is also Principal with Capital Health Advisors LLC, a health care consultancy. Shiver is a seasoned health care executive and thought leader, consultant, and physician practice manager.

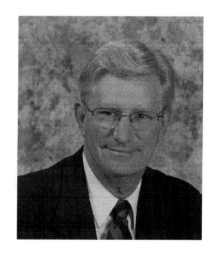

Shiver has more than 35 years of experience in hospital administration, physician practice management, teaching, and management consulting. As a consultant he has assisted health care organizations and medical universities across the country. He has advised health system leaders, boards of trustees, physicians, and medical school leaders on a broad range of issues including strategic planning, mergers and acquisitions, new venture development, strategic alliances, organizational development, conflict resolution, clinical service line development, and ambulatory care strategies.

Prior to his management consulting career, Shiver had 15 years of hospital operations experience with teaching facilities of up to 970 beds. He also served as the CEO of a 160-physician group practice and physician billing company.

Shiver has served as faculty for the American College of Healthcare Executives and the American Academy of Medical Administrators, and lectures nationally. He publishes regularly, has edited numerous texts and newsletters, hosted health care Internet sites, and hosted a television show.

Shiver earned his master's in hospital administration (MHA) from Virginia Commonwealth University Medical College of Virginia and received a bachelor's of science (BS) from The Citadel. He has served as past president of National Capital Healthcare Executives, past board member of Kiwanis of Washington, DC, and the United Way of Arlington County.

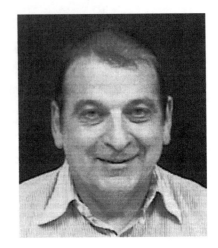

David Eitel, MD, MBA, has been involved in the clinical practice of emergency medicine for more than thirty years. He functioned as the EMRC (i.e., EMS-ALS) medical director for York and Adams Counties from 1983 to 1989, and founded the department's clinical research program in the ALS system. He was the department's first director of research from 1983 to 1998. Eitel developed the York Hospital Emergency Medicine Residency curriculum in 1988 and was the program's first residency director from 1989 to 1992. He completed a 3-year executive MBA at the Sellinger School of Business at Loyola College in Baltimore from 1993 to 1996 and became interested in operations research and the management sciences (OR/MS) during that time. Eitel is the coinventor (with the late Dr. Rich Wuerz) of the Emergency Severity Index (ESI)© triage algorithm, and a member of the ESI Triage Research Team (www.ahrq.gov/research/esi). He is chair of the Operations Management Committee of the American Academy of Emergency Medicine (AAEM), an international effort; functions as a Health Care Life Sciences consultant to the Orlando Software Group, a Microsoft partner; and is an adjunct professor in the Department of Health Administration and Policy at George Mason University in Fairfax, Virginia.

About the Contributors

Elif Akçalı received a BS degree in industrial engineering from Middle East Technical University, Ankara, Turkey, in 1990, and MS and PhD degrees in industrial engineering from Purdue University, West Lafayette, Indiana, in 1996 and 2001, respectively. She worked as a part-time consultant at Harris Semiconductor from 1996 through 1998 during her graduate studies. She is an associate professor with the Department of Industrial and Systems Engineering at the University of Florida, Gainesville. Her research interests focus on the use of mathematical programming for optimization of design and operation decisions for manufacturing programming and service systems. Her work has been published in the *Journal of Operations Management, Naval Research Logistics, IEEE Transactions*, and *International Production of Research*. She teaches courses on lean production systems, inventory and supply chain systems, and heuristic optimization. She is currently an associate editor for *IEEE Transactions on Automation Science and Engineering*.

Richard Andrews is a director of Management Engineering at Banner Health. He has 38 years of progressive health care experience in executive and consulting roles. He has provided support to approximately 1,200 hospitals and been a frequent presenter at state and national levels. His leadership, innovation, and expertise cover a broad spectrum of topics including: operational and performance improvement, decision support, information systems, advanced performance measurement and quality improvement, logistics, and materials management. He holds a BSIE and MBA from Northeastern University.

James R. Broyles is a PhD candidate in operations research at Arizona State University's Industrial Engineering Department. He has experience in manufacturing and health care engineering. His health care experience includes emergency department redesigns, outpatient clinic modeling, and facility layouts. Broyles's dissertation is focused on probability model approximations of patient throughput in hospitals.

Mary Ellen Bucco is a program director of Management Engineering at Banner Health. Her background includes 20 years in manufacturing working for companies including Eastman Kodak, Harris Corporation, and Foxboro Company.

Since arriving at Banner Health, Bucco has spent the past 3 years working with Arizona State University to bring engineering concepts into the emergency department. This work lead to an Agency for Healthcare Research and Quality (AHRQ) grant, where she co-led work with Arizona State University to develop a publicly available toolkit for improving door-to-doctor times, which includes modeling and change management tools. After implementing these tools within Banner, Bucco has shifted her focus to sharing her knowledge with hospitals throughout the country.

Twila Burdick is vice president of Organizational Performance at Banner Health, a regional health care provider with 22 hospitals in seven Western states. She provides administrative direction for departments and teams focusing on measuring and improving operational and clinical performance. In doing so, she has partnered with Arizona State University to bring high-level engineering skills to health care. She holds a master degree in business administration from the University of Montana.

Greg Butler is executive vice president for Chip Caldwell & Associates and brings more than 25 years of experience to the health care industry. During his career, Butler has held leadership positions with some of the country's leading health care manufacturers, service providers, and consulting firms. His experience includes the development of pharmacy and supply chain programs for one of the nation's largest group purchasing organizations and Cardinal Health. Butler's multifaceted background provides him with expertise to rapidly analyze client's needs and match them to applicable methods for optimizing their performance. His personal areas of expertise include: strategic planning and business plan development; client need analysis and project management; market ananlysis and consumer research; application of quality and cost reduction methodologies; and evaluation and negotiation of outsourced business agreements. He is also certified in Lean-Six Sigma and advanced quality methodologies. Butler has assisted hospitals with improving productivity and lowering operating costs for the past 15 years. He uses his experience to develop effective solutions for the many challenges facing his clients. During the past few years, his focus has been assisting clients by developing strategies for improving patient satisfaction and improving clinical utilization.

Chip Caldwell, FACHE, is president of Chip Caldwell & Associates, an innovative firm specializing in strategic deployment of Lean-Six Sigma resulting in cost position improvement, financial turnarounds, and patient throughput optimization. Chip Caldwell & Associates has helped hundreds of clients increase productivity, maximize patient throughput, and improve patient satisfaction. Caldwell is a thought leader in health care quality and performance improvement methodology. For the past decade he has served in leadership positions in the quality community including the Baldrige Foundation Board Support Team as well as the health care representative on the U.S. Quality Council. His books are widely read by hospital board members, senior leaders, middle managers, and health administration students. His more notable publications include *Mentoring Strategic Change in Health Care: An Action Guide; The Handbook for Managing Change in Healthcare; Medication Safety and Cost Recovery: A Four-Step Approach for Executives;* and *Lean-Six Sigma: An Executive Guide for Improving Cost and Patient Throughput.* Caldwell has extensive practical knowledge of hospital operations and has served in numerous leadership positions including senior vice president, Premier Performance Services; senior health industry executive, Juran Institute; president, HCA Atlanta Health System; and president/CEO, HCA West Paces Medical Center in Atlanta. Caldwell is an internationally recognized speaker and keynotes many leading conferences, including the National Patient Safety Summit, Evidence-Based Medicine Summit, Joint Commission, American Hospital Association (AHA), Institute for Healthcare Improvement, Australia Minister of Health Conference, National Healthcare Forum, and Ontario Hospital Association. He was selected by the European Organization for Quality to head the European Demonstration Project in December 1994. As a recognized author, he has served on the editorial advisory boards of the American College of Healthcare Executive's (ACHE) Health Administration Press, Aspen's Quality Management in Healthcare, Quality Progress, and the AHA's National Healthcare Forum. Caldwell is the leading executive faculty on the effective use of Lean-Six Sigma in health care for ACHE and American Society for Quality (ASQ).

Jeffery K. Cochran, PhD, is professor and head of the Department of Operational Sciences at the Air Force Institute of Technology. Cochran joined the AFIT/ENS Department after 20-plus years in the Industrial Engineering Department at Arizona State University where he founded the Health and Human Systems Laboratory. Cochran received his PhD from Purdue University. His research and teaching interests focus on optimization of stochastic models of large-scale systems including high technology manufacturing, hospital, transportation, and supply chain systems. Most recently, he has partnered with Banner Health using engineering principles to improve hospital patient flow based upon a "whole hospital" perspective. Cochran is the author of more than 100 scholarly publications and serves on 5 journal editorial boards.

Murray J. Côté, PhD, is an associate professor in the Division of Health Care Policy and Research at the University of Colorado Denver. Côté's primary research interests are in health care operations, including patient flow, capacity planning and resource management, demand forecasting, and nurse staffing and scheduling. His research findings have been published in *Decision Sciences,* the *European Journal of Operational Research, Health Care Management Science,* and *Socio-Economic Planning Sciences.* His research has received awards from the Decision Sciences Institute and the Healthcare Financial Management Association. Côté is a member of the Decision Sciences Institute (DSI), the

Institute for Operations Research and the Management Sciences (INFORMS), and the American Society for Quality (ASQ). He is a past president of the Health Applications Section of INFORMS.

Melanie L. De Grano, PhD, is a senior consultant for IBM Global Business Services in Fairfax, Virginia. She received her BS, MS, and PhD degrees in industrial engineering and operations research from Pennsylvania State University in 2002, 2004, and 2007, respectively. Her current research interests include health care engineering, simulation, and auction applications. She is a member of the Institute for Operations Research and the Management Sciences, the Institute for Industrial Engineers, and the Society for Health Systems.

Douglas B. Dotan, president and CEO of CRG Medical Inc. and the Patient Safety Organization Services Group, is the past chair of the American Society for Quality Health Care Division. He brings more than 30 years of experience in quality assessment, risk management, safety analysis, and human factors from aviation to health care, adapting the quality management knowledge and skills in aviation safety to building Web-based expert systems for the health care sector. He earned his MA in behavioral sciences/industrial and organizational psychology from the University of Houston-Clear Lake, Texas.

Shannon Elswick, FACHE, is a 33-year health care veteran currently employed as senior vice president for Orlando Health, an eight-hospital system serving Central Florida for over 90 years. Elswick also serves as president of Dr. P. Phillips Hospital, a 237-bed wholly-owned facility that sees nearly 90,000 emergency department visits per year. He is one of two Florida Hospital Association appointees to the Florida Patient Safety Corporation. He serves the University of Central Florida on the Dean's Advisory Committee for the School of Health and Public Administration and as a member of the Community Advisory Board for the Healthcare Administration program. He is a member of the eleven-county Well Florida Council and chairs the Healthcare Subcommittee of the seven-county myregion.org initiative. His service to the American College of Healthcare Executives includes appointments to the Credentials and Regent's Advisory Committees. He also serves as vice chair of the Healthcare Purchasing Alliance Inc., member of the board of Orange Indemnity LTD, and member of the editorial board for the *American Journal of Lifestyle Medicine*. Elswick has been recognized as one of the Ten Most Influential Businessmen in Central Florida by the *Orlando Business Journal*.

Tom Falvo, DO, MBA, is a graduate of the Philadelphia College of Osteopathic Medicine and the Carey School of Business at Johns Hopkins University. He completed a residency in emergency medicine (EM) at the University of Chicago in 1991. Falvo has published and lectured on the management and economics of emergency health care. He is a health care consultant and faculty member of the

EM residency program at York Hospital in York, Pennsylvania, where he directs and teaches the Business for Doctors seminar.

Ginger H. Ferguson, MN, NEA-BC, FACHE, is president of Ferguson & Associates Healthcare Consulting as well as assistant professor of nursing at Loewenberg School of Nursing, University of Memphis. She consulted with the University of Memphis in developing an Executive Nurse Leadership MSN degree program and presently serves as faculty. She is also a seasoned health care executive and leader with expertise in patient care, nursing, and clinical operations. Her expertise includes designing and implementing integrated patient care delivery systems, case management/quality management systems, automated clinical decision support and documentation systems, and redesigning emergency departments.

James Lifton, FACHE, has been in health care since 1972. He works with hospitals, health systems, and related organizations in strategy formulation, governance, business planning, and medical staff development. Lifton writes and speaks on key issues in health care management, including strategy, medical staff development, and health care system performance (including a project with American Hospital Association's (AHA) section on health care systems). He has been published in *Trustee, Health Care Strategic Management,* and *Spectrum,* and has been a faculty member for the American College of Healthcare Executives (ACHE) Congress. Lifton is a Fellow of the ACHE, where he has served on the Committee on Elections and the Regent's Advisory Council for Metropolitan Chicago. Lifton is also a certified public accountant. Lifton completed his undergraduate work at the University of Illinois, earned an MS from Wayne State University, and earned his MBA with a concentration in hospital administration from the University of Chicago.

Sueanne McKniff, RN, obtained her bachelor of science degree in nursing from York College of Pennsylvania in 1989. Since that time she has held various positions at the Department of Emergency Medicine at York Hospital–WellSpan Health System in York, Pennsylvania. Eighteen years of clinical nursing experience in the emergency department have provided a foundation as a subject matter expert of not only emergency care but also of the process inefficiencies that plague the health care system. In 2001, in addition to her nursing career, McKniff assumed the role of creative marketing director for a food packaging company. Successful throughput management of perishable food items such as chocolate and frozen spinach demand meticulous application of Lean principles. McKniff recognized the need to apply the lessons learned on the front lines of the manufacturing industry to the health care arena. Her interest on the data-driven logic behind Six Sigma peeked when she consulted with a performance improvement company. As a result, she obtained her Green Belt in Six Sigma from Drexel University in 2007. McKniff is currently employed as a clinical informatics specialist for WellSpan Health System.

Susan O'Hara, RN, BA, MPH, is the founder and president of O'Hara HealthCare Consultants LLC (OHC), a Massachusetts-based firm providing health care consulting services for hospitals, health care facilities, and architects through modeling and simulation. Through her company O'Hara has provided programming and planning services on a variety of inpatient and outpatient projects, including perioperative services, pain management, hematology/oncology, mammography, nuclear medicine, cardiac rehabilitation, invasive labs, outpatient clinics, and psychiatry. O'Hara's early simulation modeling services on the ambulatory surgery prep and recovery unit designed by Mark Sullivan Architects was featured in the textbook *Operations Research*, 2nd edition (Wiley, 2005). O'Hara provided the simulation modeling team for the National Nurses Time and Motion Study led by principal investigators Ann Hendrich and Marilyn Chow. O'Hara's team completed an inpatient medical surgical unit agent-based model using nurse agents and alternative floor plans, and have begun adding patient agents to their current work. Simulation models have been created for cardiovascular, emergency, and surgical care suites as well as outpatient services. In July 2008, O'Hara cochaired, along with Charles McLean, the National Institute of Standards and Technology (NIST) Symposium "Modeling and Simulation for Emergency Management and Healthcare Systems." O'Hara graduated from St. Joseph's School of Nursing in Syracuse, New York, and earned a bachelor of arts degree from the State University of New York at Oswego, and a master of public health degree from the University of Connecticut.

Frank Overfelt is a 32-year veteran of developing staffing requirements for all hospital departments, including the emergency department. He has been national vice president of Healthcare Information and Management Systems Society (HIMSS), senior manager with KPMG, director of Management Engineering with Intermountain Healthcare, and manager of Management Engineering for Kaiser Permanente in Southern California. Overfelt has been the driving force within HIMSS to use properly engineered staffing ratios rather than legislatively mandated fixed ratios to staff all nursing venues.

Yasar A. Ozcan, PhD, is a professor of health administration at Virginia Commonwealth University. His recently authored books include *Quantitative Methods in Health Care Management* (Jossey-Bass/Wiley) and *Health Care Benchmarking and Performance Evaluation* (Springer). He is editor-in-chief of the *Journal of Health Care Management Science* and past president of Health Care Applications Section of the Institute for Operations Research and the Management Sciences.

Kevin T. Roche completed his PhD in industrial engineering from Arizona State University's Ira A. Fulton School of Engineering in August 2008. He is currently a Management Engineering director with Banner Health in Phoenix. His research has focused on issues such as capacity modeling and control in hospitals. Along with Jeffery Cochran, he has been working on developing and applying industrial engineering and operations research tools and thinking to solve problems in many aspects of the health care system.

Marlene A. Smith, PhD, is an associate professor of quantitative methods in the Business School at the University of Colorado Denver. Her research interests include econometric model selection, statistical issues in human resources management, and evaluation and measurement of business education. Her research articles have appeared in the *Journal of Statistical Computation and Simulation, Communications in Statistics: Computation and Simulation, Journal of Econometrics, Journal of Applied Econometrics, Economic Letters, Personnel Psychology,* and the *Southern Economic Journal.*

Pierce Story is an expert in dynamic process analytics, process design, strategic operations planning, and health care process simulation applications. He brings nearly 20 years of health care experience from a variety of roles, responsibilities, and applications. During his career, Story has dealt with complex process redesign, operations and performance improvement, and new construction operations analysis in many major hospital departments, including emergency and trauma services, surgical services, inpatient units, catheterization lab, and radiology, using a variety of tools, simulations, and methodologies. His most recent work is in the development of Web-based simulation applications for the dynamic management of hospital capacity, patient flow, and resource allocations. Story is trained in Six Sigma and Lean methodologies, and has taught several courses on the uses of simulation in health care applications. Story is also the current president of the Society for Health Systems, an organization of over 950 health care performance improvement specialists and engineers devoted to improvement and change, and is active in the American Society for Quality (ASQ), Healthcare Information and Management Systems Society (HIMSS), and other health care societies.

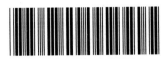